If in Doubt

If in Doubt, Breathe Out!

Breathing and support for singing
based on the Accent Method

Ron Morris and Linda Hutchison

compton
PUBLISHING

Compton Publishing

This edition first published 2017 © 2017 by Compton Publishing Ltd.

Registered office: Compton Publishing Ltd, 30 St. Giles', Oxford, OX1 3LE, UK

Registered company number: 07831037

Editorial offices: 35 East Street, Braunton, EX33 2EA, UK

Web: www.comptonpublishing.co.uk

ISBN 978-1-909082-16-8

A catalogue record for this book is available from the British Library.

Cover design: David Siddall, http://www.davidsiddall.com

Set in 11pt Adobe Caslon Pro by Regent Typesetting

1   2016

Dedication

We would like to dedicate our book to all those people who use breath, for speaking, singing or playing a musical instrument. We are nothing without breath!

Acknowledgements

There are many people who encourage, support and assist in a project like this and we are grateful to all of them. But, considering our subject, we acknowledge and thank those who set us off on the path of Accent Method in the first place: Kirsten Thyme-Frøkjær, Sara Harris, Ingrid Rugheimer and Dinah Harris. They were the people who introduced us to Accent Method, gave us the practical knowledge and encouraged us to teach and explore the method in our own work.

The idea for this book came about as a result of Ron Morris' doctoral research and he would like to acknowledge the teaching and support he received from Janice Chapman. Her pedagogy helped shape the use of Accent Method for his research.

A special thank you has to be said to Luke, Karina, Fode, Steffan, Will, Shubham and Camille, pictured in this book, for allowing Liam Harris to wander with his camera and capture them in action.

We would also like to make special mention of our colleague Ghislaine Morgan whose often heard cry "if in doubt, breathe out" to her students, workshop participants and choirs we stole (with her permission) to be the title of our book.

Finally, we acknowledge all our colleagues and students who have helped us experiment, evaluate, research and modify the use of Accent Method during the past two decades. Through you, we have arrived at a place where we feel able to share our thoughts, ideas and exercises. We hope you find them of use.

Contents

Foreword by Janice Chapman, OAM, FGS   xi

Foreword by Sara Harris, FRCSLT   xiii

Introduction and history to the Accent Method   xv

  1. Respiratory anatomy and physiology   1

  2. Breathing for singing   23

  3. Accent Method principles and practice: speaking voice   69

  4. Modifications to the Accent Method for singing   88

  5. Research into accent method for the singing voice   91

  6. The Accent method: the first steps   112

  7. The first accent bounce   121

  8. Rhythmic patterns   126

  9. Exercises into singing   132

10. A 10 week course for group teaching   137

Bibliography   150

About the Authors   155

Foreword by Janice Chapman

Accent Method has underpinned much of my vocal pedagogy. It is based securely on the body's natural respiratory patterns and clarifies and enhances a singer's ability to connect to the natural support system which is part of primal sound.

Accent Method exercises work as a means of training a singer in good effective breath management to a gold standard. Where there have been vocal problems it is a unique remedial tool. Singers are able to practise their breathing exercises separately from their repertoire to lay down healthy natural breath support.

Ron and Linda have carefully laid out the sequence of the exercises and the reasoning behind them. The teaching of Accent Method is clearly and concisely explained throughout and readers are able to choose how much of the underpinning scientific information they wish to read.

I thoroughly recommend this valuable addition to Vocal Pedagogy.

Professor Janice L. Chapman, OAM, FGS
Guildhall School of Music and Drama, London

Foreword by Sara Harris

'To breathe or not to breathe' has been the title of many a lecture over recent years. At last we have a guide: *If in Doubt, Breathe Out!* The area of breathing as applied to singing pedagogy has frequently been controversial. There have been a variety of interesting and sometimes strange theories about breathing and singing, and the topic always produces plenty of lively discussion between voice practitioners. It is therefore very refreshing to see collaboration between a singing teacher and a speech and language pathologist that approaches this shared area of interest in a pragmatic and evidence based way.

The approach the authors take is founded on the principles and practices of the 'Accent Method', a technique developed in Denmark by Phonetician Svend Smith between 1935 and 1970. The technique was further developed by Danish speech and language therapist Kirsten Thyme-Frøkjær who, along with other more recent practitioners, carried out the research that makes Accent Method one of the few voice techniques to have a sound, level 1 evidence base. In the past, Accent Method has been used successfully to treat stammerers and those with voice disorders. It has also been shown to be valuable in developing effective voicing for normal speakers and has been used regularly to train the voices of undergraduate speech and language therapists in Sweden. However, although there was considerable anecdotal evidence, there was no hard evidence to show Accent breathing was also effective for developing flexible breath control in singers. The research carried out in Ron Morris's doctoral thesis has now provided that much needed evidence and has also validated the work of those of us already devoted to working on Accent Method with singers.

Linda Hutchison and Ron Morris are both distinguished and well known names in the worlds of singing teaching and voice therapy, each with a wealth of practical experience and expertise developed during their respective careers. This book is a coming together of that knowledge, experience and research as applied to the area of breathing. The authors show us in an engaging way, how an understanding of the anatomy and physiology of breathing can help us find our way through the plethora of ideas and exercises out there in the field so we can 'home in' on those that work the best. They provide numerous little gems of insight along with the easy to follow practical exercises that are presented and illustrated in the text. Throughout the book there is a clear, theoretical underpinning to show why these exercises work.

If in Doubt, Breath Out! will prove invaluable for those already working as singing teachers, those who are developing their skills to become singing teachers and to singers who want a better understanding of how their breathing works. It will also be immensely helpful to speech and language therapists working in the area of voice disorder, particularly when they come across performers in trouble, and to speech therapy students new to the area of voice and the needs of performers. It is hoped that *If in Doubt, Breath Out!* will demystify breathing for speakers and singers for generations to come.

Sara Harris, FRCSLT
Specialist Speech and Language Therapist (Voice), Lewisham Voice Clinic, Lewisham Hospital, London and Past-President, The British Voice Association

Introduction and history of the Accent Method

The Accent Method in its original form comes from the world of therapeutic voice. There has been a great deal of research done showing how effective it is for the speaking voice. Towards the end of the 20th century, Accent Method began to be embraced, absorbed and adapted into a valuable tool for the singer and the singing studio. There was, however, no research focussing specifically on the singing voice. The first scientific data came in Ron Morris' doctoral thesis which looked at the Method's effects on the singing voice. This confirmed what we were finding in practice and instinctively felt to be true: Accent Method with the necessary adjustments for singing is as effective for the singing voice as it has proved for the speaking voice over these many decades.

Accent Method started life as *Svend Smith's Method of Voice Training* (Thyme-Frøkjær and Frøkjær-Jensen, 2001, p. 6) in the 1930s. At that time Svend Smith, a voice physiologist and clinician, was director of the Experimental Phonetics Laboratory, part of the Institute of Voice Disorders at Hellerup, Denmark. He was in the position of being able to look at things scientifically as well as from the practical point of view. This underpins the strength of the Accent Method: sound in science, effective in practice.

Professor Smith felt there was a need for a practical voice training programme which could be used safely and effectively, particularly on damaged and fragile voices. The various methods of voice training around at the time were aimed more at relatively healthy voices. As a result, they were not very successful in helping to restore an injured voice, or a pathologically disordered voice. It should be noted that Accent Method can also be used as a therapeutic tool for working with people who stutter or stammer.

Svend Smith researched extensively the voice training systems of the nineteenth and early twentieth centuries, as well as the physics of how the vocal folds work. Experiments he undertook showed the aerodynamic and myoelastic behaviour of the folds, which is still the basis for the current theory on how the vocal folds vibrate to make sound.

By 1937, he had put together his findings and drawn up a plan of action for treatment. However, there was to be an interesting add-on a year later which, perhaps, was a sign all those years ago that this was eventually going to be a good thing for the singing world! Smith attended what has been described as a 'jam' session in Copenhagen (Thyme-Frøkjær and Frøkjær-Jensen, 2001, p. 6). The performer at this particular gig was the American-born (later French citizen) dancer, singer and actress, Josephine Baker. There is no record as to what Svend thought of *her*, but he obviously was fascinated by the bongo playing of Bogano, Miss Baker's drummer. The two men got together later and from that meeting, a set of drum exercises was added to the voice training system.

From then on, all the theoretical work could be put into practice. This he did with his own patients. However, he continued to test his results through the years in order to show scientifically that the exercises were indeed achieving what was intended.

In 1967, a speech and language therapist, Kirsten Thyme-Frøkjær began to collaborate with Smith in his research. This was to lead to further development of the *Svend Smith's Method of Voice Training*. And it was at this point that it was decided to change the name. The new name would highlight the important feature of the stresses, or accents, in the rhythmic exercises. And so, from then on it became known as The Accent Method.

Svend Smith became Professor of Phonetics at Hamburg University in 1969. He continued to organise courses in The Accent Method throughout Europe, along with several professional colleagues who had learned directly from him. *Accentmetoden*, the first book to give the theory, the exercises and how these transferred into day-to-day speaking was co-authored in 1978 with Kirsten Thyme-Frøkjær.

Professor Smith died in 1985. Happily, the work he pioneered continues thanks to the many practitioners, notably Kirsten Thyme-Frøkjær and Børge Frøkjær-Jensen, who continue to research, write about and promote Accent Method.

As with all systems and methods, the work gets moulded and subtly altered in the hands of different practitioners. However, the principles remain; We cannot stress enough how vital it is to understand these principles and the philosophy behind the method

Ron Morris, Ph.D.
Linda Hutchison

1

Respiratory anatomy and physiology

To a great extent, modern scientific methods, particularly in the last 50 years, have enabled us to understand how the voice and breathing mechanisms operate. As use of the flexible fibreoptic nasendoscope became more common from the late 1970s, much of the research into the voice has focused on the larynx and the movement of the vocal folds, with little attention being given to breathing and support. However, some work has been directed towards breath management and support systems.

Apart from the study of singing, a lot of work into the respiratory system and breath management has been carried out by physiologists, speech pathologists, physiotherapists and respiratory physicians. Many of these studies have focused on how the structures and muscles of the respiratory system work and interact in live subjects. This information has allowed us to move beyond that derived from cadavers in the anatomy rooms, or from the sensations of the singers themselves.

The study of anatomy is vital to understand the structure of the body, i.e. 'the respiratory system'. However, anatomy alone cannot provide completely accurate information about how those structures operate and particularly, how they interact when performing specific tasks. The science of respiratory physiology is complex, but a solid understanding is very helpful for the singer and singing teacher. This said, there are a number of core concepts which, if mastered, allow the singer and teacher to work effectively with breath management.

Core concepts in respiratory anatomy and physiology

Air moves from areas of high pressure to areas of low pressure

- When a person breathes in, extra space is created in the chest cavity, which means that the air pressures in the lungs drop. As the pressure in the lungs is now lower than that of the outside air, the air will move into the body and fill the lungs. We inhale!

The primary muscles for inhalation are the diaphragm and the intercostal muscles.

- As the diaphragm contracts it moves downwards and forwards, opening the lower ribs and creating more space in the chest cavity which allows the lungs to fill with air. The intercostal muscles are also active during inhalation as they maintain the shape of the ribcage and prevent collapse.

- There are secondary muscles of inhalation in the shoulders, neck and back but use of these muscles can lead to excessive tension in the vocal tract, which is not conducive to good singing.

- The diaphragm is responsible for up to 80% of the volume of air breathed in during a deep breath.

- Inhalation takes about a second.

Exhalation (breathing out) can be either passive or active

- In passive exhalation, the diaphragm stops contracting and slowly returns to its resting positon. The intercostal muscles also tend to relax and the system returns to rest through elastic recoil. As the system returns to rest, the pressure in the lungs rises above that of the outside air so the air flows out. We exhale!

- In active exhalation we take control of the air either by slowing down its exit from the lungs or controlling the rate or pressure under which it leaves the lungs. Speaking, blowing, coughing, laughing or singing all require active exhalation. Active exhalation requires the use of additional muscles to control the pressure and flow of the air. Specifically, we use the abdominal muscles to do this. It may seem counter-intuitive, but if we want to actively exhale, slow down the rate of the air leaving the body, we engage the abdominal muscles to help us breathe out. The chest wall is well supplied with mechano-pressure receptors which send a signal to the brainstem to tell the respiratory centre what is occurring within the lungs in terms of air pressure and volume. When the pressures are higher, the respiratory centre tells the intercostal muscles and the diaphragm to maintain their activity (i.e., breathe in), which acts like a releasing brake and slows down the exit of air from the lungs. As we engage our abdominal muscles to help us breathe out, the lung pressures are high for a much longer time, encouraging the diaphragm and intercostal muscles to remain active and hence slow the air flow down. In more explosive gestures, such as coughing or sneezing, the air exits the lungs in a huge rush, showing what happens when we engage the abdominal muscles to breathe out, but do not operate the inhalatory muscles to act as brakes.

- Timing of actions and co-ordination of the whole respiratory system is required for specific tasks. Speaking or singing requires a different respiratory organisation to coughing or sneezing for example.

- Passive exhalation takes about twice as long as inhalation (i.e., about two seconds).

- Active exhalation can be slowed so that it becomes up to 20 or 30 times longer than inhalation (i.e. 20 to 30 seconds).

- Muscles can only contract (shorten) or relax (return to their resting state); they cannot expand although they can be stretched by other muscles.

If you would like to know more of the science behind the respiratory system, including the musculature, please read on. The next section can be omitted as long as you understand the core concepts listed above as they are vital to the understanding of how Accent Method breathing works and can be used.

Scary science component begins now!

The structure and function of the respiratory system

The respiratory system (Figure 1.1) is a complex arrangement of structures that has as its primary goal the exchange of air. Oxygen is taken on board by the body and waste carbon dioxide is expelled through the auspices of the respiratory system. Hixon (1987) reminds us that the human respiratory system has two main functions: breathing for life and breathing for speech or singing.

The respiratory system consists of

- a set of tubes that connect the lungs to the outside air (the trachea, bronchi and bronchioles)

- the lungs, where gas exchange occurs

- the ribcage, which serves to both protect the delicate lungs and assist in their management

- muscular structures that provide the necessary energy to drive the system.

The respiratory system is predominantly housed in the thorax (chest), but a number of its muscular components are contained in the abdomen and also attach to the back.

The tubes that connect the respiratory system to the outside air are generally considered to begin below the level of the larynx. The larynx (voice box) acts as a valve that prevents food and fluid from the pharynx (throat) entering the airway. Above the level of the larynx, in the mouth and pharynx, air and food share a common pathway. Interestingly, the nose, which has a major function in warming and humidifying the air we breathe, is used only by air. There is no significant difference in breathing through the mouth or through the nose in terms of how respiration works, but nasal breathing tends to be slower.

The trachea runs from the lower border of the larynx (at about the level of the fifth cervical vertebra) to opposite the third thoracic vertebra where it divides into two bronchi, one for each lung. The trachea is essentially a cylinder made up of cartilage and membrane. The cylinder is slightly flattened at the posterior aspect (towards the back). There are between 16 and 20 segments (known as the tracheal rings) in the trachea which look like irregularly shaped rings; the anterior portion (towards the front) is cartilage and the posterior portion is made up of a fibrous membrane which is a flexible wall shared with the oesophagus. The entire structure is enclosed in a fibrous but elastic membrane. Leonard (1983) informs us that the male adult trachea is approximately 11–12 cm in length and 2–2.5 cm in diameter (in females the tracheal diameter may be slightly smaller). There is some variation in the number of tracheal rings, the number of rings in each bronchus and the exact diameter of the rings from person to person.

The right bronchus is approximately 2.5 cm long and is made up of six to nine rings. It is shorter and at a more horizontal angle than the left bronchus. The bronchus continues to divide (these divisions are known as bronchioles) until the alveoli are reached. The alveoli are the air cells where exchange of gases occurs; they are very small and are lined with delicate mucous membrane.

The left bronchus is longer than the right, being approximately 5 cm in length. It has nine to 12 rings and is of a slightly smaller diameter. The left bronchus, on its journey to the lung, has to cross the oesophagus and the descending aorta; it also continues to divide into bronchioles until the alveoli are reached.

The lungs are often simply defined as a pair of spongy sacs. Hixon (1987) describes them as 'cone shaped structures that are of a porous, spongy texture and that possess an abundance of resilient elastic fibres.' (p. 6). He goes on to say that whilst it is a gross over-simplification of their structure and function, there is some value in seeing the lungs as large elastic sacs that are filled with air and which have the ability to change size and shape (Hixon, 1987, p. 6).

The right lung is slightly larger than the left, having three lobes instead of two. This is due to the fact that the heart and lungs share the thoracic cavity and the heart is, of course, situated to the left.

The lungs are covered with membranes known as the visceral pleura. There is also a pleural (known as the parietal pleura) lining to the thoracic cavity and the top of the diaphragm. 'Together these membranes form a double walled sac that completely encases the lungs. Both walls of this sac are covered with a thin layer of lubricating fluid that permits them to move easily one on another' (Hixon, 1987, p. 7). Rubin (1998) states that 'the pleural cavity is a fluid filled potential space that binds the lungs to the ribcage and diaphragm such that any movements therein cause corresponding increases or decreases in lung volumes' (p. 51). This close relationship between the two layers of pleura and the lungs on one side, and the ribcage and diaphragm on the other, is called 'pleural linkage' and is the reason that changes in the shape of the thorax directly impact on lung volumes. As the diaphragm descends and the lower ribs are expanded, this pleural linkage ensures that the lungs also get larger which, of course, lowers the air pressure inside them.

The ribcage which bounds the area known as the thoracic cavity is described by Hixon as a barrel shaped cage of bone and cartilage. The ribcage is bounded at the back by the thoracic vertebrae which are vertebrae numbers eight to 19 (there being 34 vertebrae in man, seven cervical, 12 thoracic and 15 abdominal). The thoracic vertebrae comprise only a very small portion of the cage as most of it is formed by the ribs.

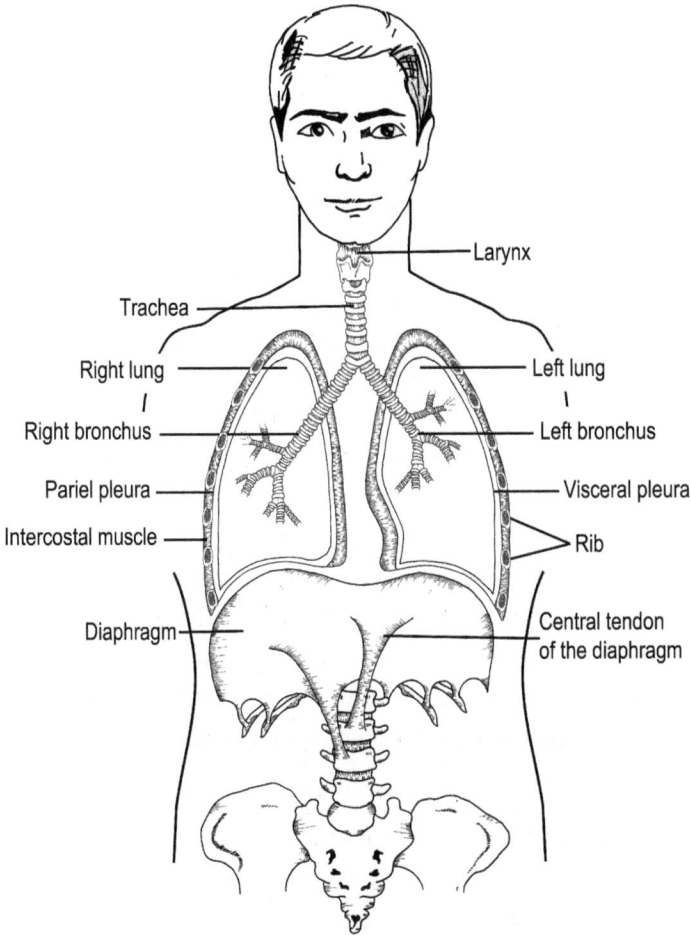

Figure 1.1 The respiratory system

There are 12 ribs, one arising from each of the thoracic vertebrae. The ribs are flat, arch-shaped bones that slope downwards and outwards to give the ribcage its characteristic rounded form. At the front, rib number one is essentially fused to the flat sternum or breast bone, while the ribs numbered two to seven have costal cartilages that join independently to the sternum. The costal cartilages from ribs number eight, nine and 10 join that of rib number seven, so they are not attached to the sternum directly. Ribs 11 and 12 are known as the floating ribs and have no attachment at their anterior ends. Because of their attachments and the arrangement of the ligament and joint capsules, the ribs are capable of movement at both their vertebral and sternal ends. The arrangement of the joint and ligaments allows the ribs to move slightly up and down on the vertebrae, and to rotate to some degree, but not to move outwards from the vertebrae. At the anterior end of the ribs the costal cartilages numbered two to seven all have joints to the sternum that allow movement.

The first rib is the shortest, after which rib length increases until rib seven after which it decreases. The length and orientation of the ribs determine the pattern of movement which they demonstrate. Bunch (1997) states that the ribs can be described as having both a pump handle and a bucket handle movement (Figure 1.2). Ribs one to five are usually described as having the pump handle motion. In these ribs, the most lateral part of the rib tends to be lower in relation to the vertebral and sternal ends so that the sternal end moves obliquely on inspiration, thus increasing the anterior–posterior dimensions of the chest. Ribs numbers five to 10, on inspiration, tend to move the chest wall in a lateral as well as in an anterior–posterior direction and are thus described as having a bucket handle motion.

Many singing pedagogies ascribe great importance to the movement of the ribs in breath management but it is interesting to note that Bunch, in her 1997 text *Dynamics of the singing voice*, takes great pains to describe the exact nature of the ribs and their movement but asserts that 'the well-trained singer does not move these [ribs numbers one to five] very much for two reasons; (1) the diaphragm plays a major role in their breathing pattern and (2) the ribcage is already partially elevated by the assumption of the correct posture.' (p. 35). Bunch (1997) also states that excessive movement of these ribs is detrimental to good singing because it usually requires the use of neck muscles. Additional and unwanted tension around the larynx can be created by the excessive use of the neck muscles in singing:

The dimensions of the chest cavity can be increased in a number of planes due to the movement of the ribs. The lower ribs 5, 6 and 7, and due to the connection of the costal cartilages ribs 8, 9 and 10, participate most in this movement. 'When the body is properly aligned, these natural movements of the lower chest and abdomen become obvious both to the singer and the trained observer.' (Bunch, 1997, p36)

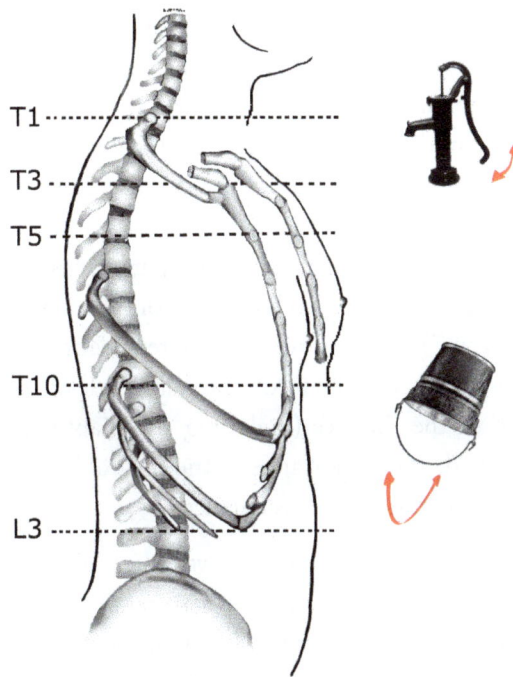

Figure 1.2 Pump handle action of the ribs. Image from Harris and Howard: *Voice Clinic Handbook* 2edn, Compton Publishing, 2017.

The muscles that drive the respiratory system can be found in both the thorax and the abdomen and they act on the lungs not directly, but through the binding of the lungs to the ribcage and diaphragm that occurs via the visceral and parietal pleurae. The respiratory system is flexible and elastic throughout and the muscular forces that operate on it do so against this backdrop of stretch and recoil. Singers and teachers need to understand that there are a number of forces that operate on the lungs to help control and manage airflow and pressure.

Hixon (1987) states that 'Although the lungs and the thorax normally operate together as a unit, it is important to realise that their natural resting positions in the intact unit are different from their individual resting positions when the two are separated'. If the lungs were to be removed from the thorax they would immediately collapse and contain almost no air. The elastic tissues of the bronchioles and alveoli would spring back to their smallest state so that they would be of a significantly smaller volume. The resting position of the thorax with the lungs removed is more expanded and would be of a greater volume (Hixon, 1987, Sundberg, 1987). 'With the lungs and thorax held together as a unit by pleural linkage, the respiratory apparatus assumes a resting position between these two separate positions such that the lungs are somewhat expanded and the thorax is somewhat compressed' (Hixon, 1987, p.7). This resting position represents a state of balance or a neutral position where the force of the lungs' desire to collapse is equal to the force of the thorax's (including the diaphragm and abdomen) desire to expand. The importance of the pleural linkage cannot be over emphasised in maintaining this balance.

The pressures within the respiratory system are also of great importance to the understanding of how the respiratory musculature operates. Pressure can be identified within the lungs (alveolar pressure), between the two pleural walls that are within the thorax but outside the lungs (pleural pressure), and within the abdomen (abdominal pressure). Pleural pressure tends to be a constant as it is the pressure between the two layers of pleura. Alveolar pressure and abdominal pressure vary much more and it is these variations in pressure that allow us to breathe. It is important to remember that with the respiratory apparatus in the resting position, alveolar pressure is equal to atmospheric pressure. This resting position occurs for brief and transient periods of time in the respiratory cycle, unless of course the subject has died and respiration has ceased!

The mechanics and function of respiration relate directly to the muscles that drive the system. It can be viewed in terms of the breath cycle, inhalation and exhalation, and in terms of the volumes and pressures within the respiratory system.

Inhalation

Inhalation (or inspiration) occurs when air flows into the lungs. 'Air flows from regions of higher pressure to regions of lower pressure' (Hixon, 1987, p. 8). Should the airways be open and the respiratory system in neutral or resting position, there would be no flow as the alveolar pressure is equal to the atmospheric pressure. To achieve air movement into the lungs the alveolar pressure must be lowered so that it is lower than the atmospheric pressure, causing air to flow into the lungs.

Boyle's Law states that pressure and volume are inversely proportional to each other. This means that when the volume is increased the pressure is decreased, and when the volume is decreased the pressure is increased. Pressure (in the respiratory system) occurs when the air molecules in the lungs collide with each other.

Decreased alveolar pressure is achieved by increasing the volume of the lungs. Since the lungs are linked to the thoracic cavity by the pleural linkage, increases in thoracic volume result in increases in lung volume, decreases in alveolar pressure and the subsequent inward flow of air.

The muscles that increase the volume of the thoracic cage can be separated into two groups: the primary muscles of inspiration, consisting of the diaphragm and the intercostal muscles; and the accessory muscles of inspiration such as the sternocleidomastoid, scalenes, pectoralis minor, serratus anterior, serratus posterior, quadratus lumborum and levatores costarum. Some writers also include the pectoralis major, the subclavius and the latissimus dorsi as accessory muscles of inspiration, but as their role appears to be only in very forced respiration and indeed under

11

some dispute, they can be ignored for the purposes of this discussion. Campbell (1970) goes so far as to state that 'of all the muscles which are generally thought to act as accessory muscles of inspiration, only the scaleni and the sternomastoids [sternocleidomastoids] show significant respiratory activity in man' (p. 181). These muscles act to lift the ribcage directly, usually by lifting the shoulders and achieving a limited amount of increase in the size of the thoracic cavity.

The diaphragm is a large, double-domed muscle which attaches to the back of the xiphoid process, the inner surfaces of the costal cartilages seven to 12, and the vertebral column. At rest, the right side is slightly higher than the left and the diaphragm has a depressed space towards the centre where the heart lies. The diaphragm is always active in inspiration regardless of the type of inspiration, and Bunch (1997, p. 37) states that 'it is responsible for 60–80% of increased volume in deep inspiration'.

When the diaphragm is activated its fibres shorten and straighten, causing the domes to descend. The diaphragm therefore flattens and comes forward, pushing the contents of the abdomen slightly down and out. The muscles of the abdomen yield to this increased abdominal pressure causing an outward bulge in the upper abdomen (epigastrium). This in turn increases the vertical depth of the thoracic cavity. The diaphragm also attaches to the lower ribs so as it descends, these are pulled gently outwards (open) which creates additional space within the thoracic cavity laterally. Some singers and teachers actually believe that the bulging out at the epigastrium is the diaphragm itself! This bulge is caused by the action of the diaphragm but the diaphragm itself cannot be readily felt or palpated.

Electrical activity of the diaphragm has been studied using needle electrodes through the costal part of the body wall, or using bipolar surface electrodes placed in the oesophagus.

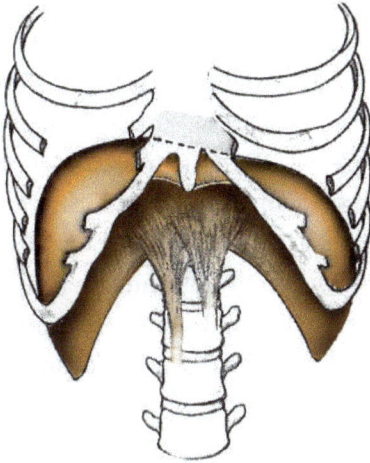

Figure 1.3 Anterior view of the Diaphragm. Image from Harris and Howard: *Voice Clinic Handbook* 2edn, Compton Publishing, 2017.

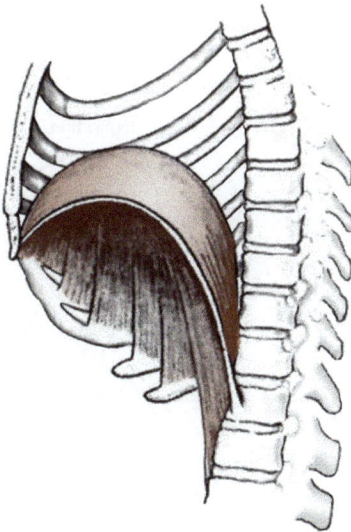

Figure 1.4 Sagittal section showing the right hemidiaphragm from the left. Image from Harris and Howard: *Voice Clinic Handbook* 2edn, Compton Publishing, 2017.

'During quiet breathing the (electrical) activity increases progressively throughout inspiration and decreases in the early part of expiration to become nil at about half the expiration time'(Agostoni & Sant Ambrogio, 1970, p.152). The diaphragm is also active during expulsive efforts such as parturition, defaecation or vomiting, during which activities it works synergistically with the abdominal muscles to increase intra-abdominal pressure. Some activity is also found during strong expiratory efforts, particularly when lung volumes are low. During phonation the diaphragm's activity diminishes and ceases during the first two to three seconds after inspiration (Agostoni & Sant Ambrogio, 1970, p.154). The diaphragm's role during the expiration phase in classical singing is under dispute. However, Sundberg (1987) reports a study where the diaphragm was active under a number of conditions during the expiration phase, and Bouhuys, Proctor and Mead (1966) found that three out of five non-professional singers use active diaphragm activity to balance the respiratory recoil forces at high lung volumes. It appears that the diaphragm may have a role to play in balancing the pneumatic forces in the respiratory system during singing. In fact, we know that when lung volumes are high the diaphragm, along with the intercostal muscles, acts like a releasing brake to control the exit of air from the lungs. This respiratory control appears to be driven by breath pressure rather than conscious thought.

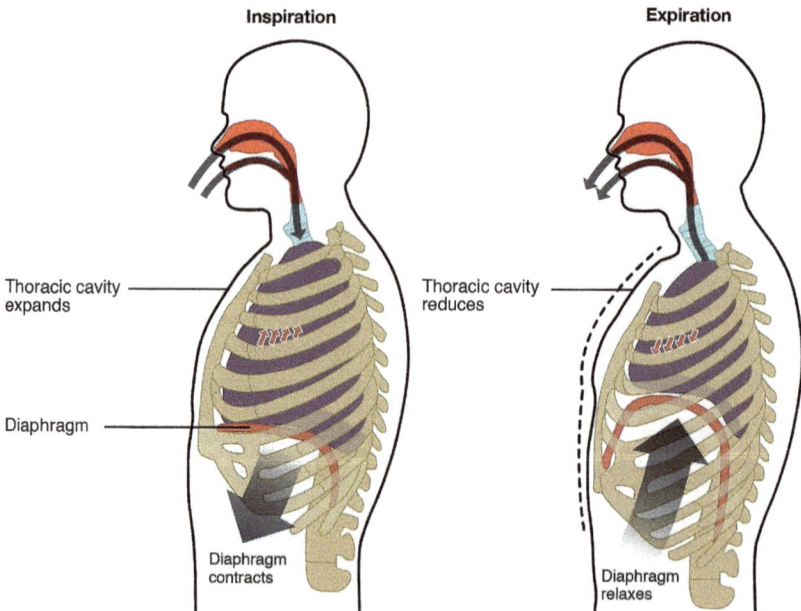

Figure 1.5 Diagram showing the effects of diaphragmatic descent. Courtesy of OpenStax College, Creative Commons license, via Wikimedia Commons

The intercostal muscles are actually found in three layers lying between the ribs. These are known as the external and internal intercostals, with a third, internal layer known as the innermost intercostals.

The external intercostals extend from the inferior margin of one rib to the superior margin of the one below, with the muscle fibres running in an oblique direction oriented forward and down. Activation of the external intercostals tends to raise the ribs but because of their orientation, they work most effectively on the lower ribs (Rubin, 1998, p. 54). Bunch (1997, p. 39) disagrees with this statement as she feels that most rib raising occurs through diaphragm action, with the external intercostal muscles serving only to stabilise the ribcage wall to allow the diaphragm to move the ribs as a unit. Bunch (1997, p. 39) also points out that much of the literature on intercostal muscle function in books on speech and voice is not up-to–date, and she sets out a useful review of the literature on the function of the intercostal muscles.

As early as the 1950s, Campbell attempted to study the electrical activity of the respiratory muscles using surface electrodes. 'He concluded that some parts of the intercostals were active in quiet inspiration and in voluntary forced inspiration, and that no distinction was possible between the internal and external layers.' (Bunch, 1997, p.39). Taylor, in 1963, used specially constructed needle electrodes that were inserted directly into the muscles and his study used 80 human subjects. 'Taylor demonstrated two functionally distinct layers of intercostal muscle in all parts of the chest wall. The superficial one was activated only by inspiratory efforts, and the deeper one by expiratory efforts' (Bunch, 1997, p. 39).

The external intercostals are certainly active during inspiration. Whether this activation does lift the ribs themselves or merely stabilises the ribcage wall so that other (probably diaphragmatic) forces can lift it is still open to debate. Rubin (1998), Hixon (1987) and Bunch (1997) all report that the role of the intercostal muscles as a group is to stabilise the chest wall. 'Their function [the intercostal muscles] is to maintain the stability of the chest wall, to prevent it being sucked in during inspiration.' (Rubin, 1998, p. 54).

The internal and innermost intercostals lie deep to the external intercostals and their fibres run in the opposite oblique direction. Their attachments are also different; the upper attachment is further from the fulcrum of rib movement than the lower, which reverses the direction of their pull, so they are thought to lower the ribs (Rubin, 1998, p. 57). They appear to be more involved in expiration than inspiration so their actions will be discussed in more detail in the description of expiration.

During quiet respiration and much of respiration for speech, the action of the diaphragm and intercostal muscles account for most of the changes in thoracic cage dimensions. Other accessory muscles have the potential to change the size of the thoracic cage, and their use is often seen in forced inspiration or in the breathing patterns of patients who need to use an upper chest or clavicular breath pattern of breathing to compensate for paralysis or weakness in the chest muscles or diaphragm (Hixon 1987, Campbell and Newsom Davis, 1970).

Whilst these accessory muscles can be used for inspiration, reliance on them rather than on the diaphragm and intercostal muscles would be detrimental to the singer and should be discouraged as they significantly increase neck and shoulder tension even though they do create some additional space in the thoracic cavity.

Exhalation

Exhalation (or expiration) occurs when air flows from the lungs. Just as in inspiration, there has to be a difference between the alveolar pressure and atmospheric pressure if air flow is to occur. In inspiration, the alveolar pressure was dropped by increasing the lung volumes. Once inspiration has ceased, i.e., the lungs can increase in volume no more, the alveolar pressure and the atmospheric pressure will again be equal. To start the outward flow of air the alveolar pressure needs to be greater than the atmospheric pressure. 'In the human respiratory pump. this is accomplished at times by non-muscular forces and at other times by both muscular and non-muscular forces, which reduce the size of the lungs–thorax unit, thereby compressing the alveolar air and raising its pressure above atmosphere' (Hixon 1987, p. 17). In quiet respiration the expiration forces are essentially passive and consist of the elastic recoil mechanism of the lungs and ribcage (Hixon 1987, Rubin 1998 and Sundberg 1987). Thus, the movement of approximately 500 ml of air in quiet respiration is controlled predominantly by the active contraction of the diaphragm for inspiration and the elastic recoil of the system for expiration.

There are two types of expiration, passive and active, that can be employed to meet the various demands of moving air from the lungs. As stated previously passive expiration is achieved predominantly by elastic recoil of the respiratory system while active expiration requires interaction of the elastic recoil with additional muscular action.

Hixon (1987) states that 'expiration above the resting expiratory level usually is passive. As such it is accomplished not by muscular effort, but by non-muscular forces that return the lungs and the thorax to their usual volumes at the resting expiratory level' (p. 19). After quiet inspiration, when the inspiratory muscles are relaxed, the lungs will recoil towards a smaller volume. The recoiling lungs also pull inwards on the thorax and pull upwards on the diaphragm, thus reducing the size of the thoracic cavity towards neutral (resting expiratory level). It is simplistic to think that the inspiratory muscles switch off immediately that inspiration has occurred. Hixon (1987) states that: 'They [the inspiratory muscles] actually continue their activity into the early part of expiration, with the force they exert gradually decreasing and acting as a releasing brake against the lung recoil forces' (p. 19. Although this type of expiration is labelled as passive expiration, it is not truly passive until the inspiratory muscle forces switch off from their braking function at about the 2nd second in the expiration cycle.

Active expiration can occur at any time in the expiration cycle and it is not merely limited to the expiration that occurs once elastic recoil is complete. Rubin (1998, p. 57) states that active expiration is required once the lungs are at 35% vital capacity, since this is the level that is thought to be the resting expiratory level. Active expiration above this level (35% vital capacity) will serve to increase alveolar pressure and airflow, but any expiration below this level will, by necessity, be active. Rubin (1998) also states that 'for controlled expiration during phonation and for increasing the intensity or duration of sound, activities that are critical in singing, more expiratory muscular activity is necessary that that obtained via recoil' (p. 58).

Muscles of active expiration either lower the ribs or sternum to decrease the dimensions of the thorax, or increase the abdominal pressure to push the diaphragm upwards to decrease the vertical dimensions of the thorax. It is important to remember that the abdominal cavity can be seen as a muscular bag enclosed by the diaphragm at the top and the muscles of the pelvic floor below. The abdominal muscles form the sides and front of the bag. The volume within the abdominal cavity remains basically constant (since it contains the viscera) so that when the diaphragm descends the abdominal wall, when relaxed (the most flexible component of the bag), is distended. Conversely, when the muscles of the abdominal wall contract and the diaphragm is relaxed, the contents of the abdomen are driven up into the thorax raising the intra-thoracic pressure and hence expelling air from the lungs (Rubin, 1998, p. 59).

'Whereas there are multiple muscle groups that can, under varying circumstances, be brought into play for direct or accessory assistance in inspiration, there are somewhat fewer muscle groups available for expiration.' (Rubin, 1998, p. 58). Muscles that are most likely to be involved in active expiration are thought to be: internal intercostals, external abdominal oblique, rectus abdominis, transversus thoracis, transversus abdominis, internal abdominal oblique, subcostals, sacrospinals, iliocostalis lumborum and the serratus posterior inferior (Rubin, 1998, p. 59).

The internal intercostals are thin muscles that are situated in the rib spaces lying beneath the external intercostals. Their fibres run upwards and forwards from one rib to the one above. The fibres run almost at right angles to the fibres of the external intercostals (Hixon, 1987, p. 20). The internal intercostals pull the ribs downwards and stiffen the rib interspaces (Hixon, 1987, p. 20). Rubin (1998, p. 57) indicates that 'the intercostal muscles are more active during phonation/singing wherein they help maintain the subglottic pressure.'

The external abdominal oblique arises from the lower eight ribs and runs forwards, downwards and medially to insert into the rectus sheath, linea alba and iliac crest (hip bone), and the inguinal ligament in the groin (Rubin, 1998, p. 59). 'When it contracts, the external oblique draws the lower ribs downwards and displaces the contents of the abdomen inward, thus raising the abdominal pressure.' (Hixon, 1987, p.22).

The internal abdominal oblique is another large flat muscle that lies internal and slightly more medial to the external oblique. It originates rather broadly over the whole iliac crest and inguinal ligament, and its fibres run upwards and medially to insert into the costal cartilages of the lower four ribs and the mid-line abdominal aponeurosis (linea alba). On contraction this muscle draws the lower ribs down and pulls the abdominal wall inward (Hixon, 1987, p. 23).

The transversus abdominis too originates from the iliac crest and inguinal ligament, but it also arises from the inner surfaces of the lower six costal cartilages. These fibres actually interweave somewhat with the fibres of the diaphragm and the lumbar vertebrae. The fibres run transversely to insert into the linea alba rather like a cummerbund (Rubin, 1998, p. 60). On contraction, the transversus abdominis displaces the abdominal wall inward, again raising the abdominal pressure (Hixon, 1987, p. 23). We now believe that the transversus abdominis is the prime mover in generating airflow by raising abdominal pressure. It is the deepest layer of the abdominal team and should activate first in supported airflow.

The rectus abdominis originates at the crest and symphysis of the pubis, and the fibres run upwards to insert into the xiphoid process and the fifth, sixth and seventh costal cartilages. Contraction draws the sternum down and the abdominal contents inwards (Rubin, 1998, p. 60; Hixon, 1987, p. 22).

The transversus thoracis originates from the xiphoid process and the lower portion of the sternum, and runs laterally to insert onto the costal cartilages of the second to sixth ribs (Rubin, 1998, p. 60). Contraction of this muscle tends to lower the ribs to which it attaches and has an effect of narrowing the thoracic cage (Hixon, 1987, p. 21).

The subcostals are thin strips of muscles that originate from the deep surfaces of the ribs near the vertebral column and insert into the second and third ribs, near the rib angles. Their fibres parallel those of the internal intercostals and they are thought to have similar functions (Rubin, 1998, p. 60).

The sacrospinals are a group of powerful muscles that run between the ribcage and the vertebral column. Their lumbar portion forms a lever with the lower ribs and may help to depress the lower ribs (Rubin, 1998, p. 61).

The serratus posterior inferior is located on the back. It originates from the lower thoracic and the upper lumbar vertebrae, and the fibres slant upwards to insert into the lower borders of the last four ribs. Contraction of these muscles pulls the lower ribs down (Hixon, 1987, p. 22).

The quadratus lumborum is located on the back wall of the abdominal cavity. It originates from the iliac crest and the fibres run upwards to insert into the lumbar spine and the back of the lowest rib. Its contraction is thought to depress the lowest rib (Hixon, 1987, p. 22).

As with inspiration, the exact muscular interactions required for expiration are not completely understood. Anatomists evaluate muscle movements in isolation but in the living specimen there are numerous muscular interactions that occur simultaneously. Just as the inspiratory muscles do not switch off immediately expiration commences, many of the expiratory muscles work either together or in sequence to promote the desired effect of increasing abdominal and alveolar pressure.

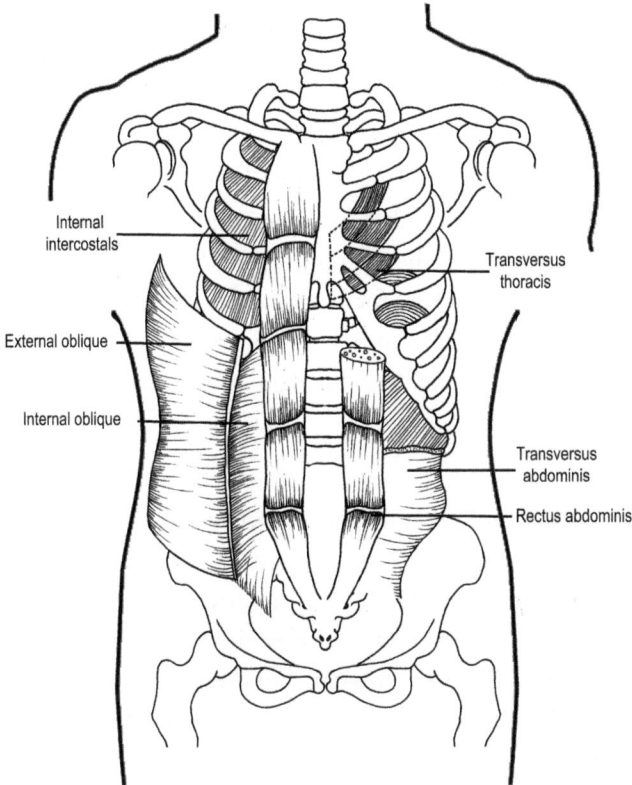

Figure 1.6 Diagram showing the muscles of expiration.

Bunch (1997, p.47) highlights the fact that these abdominal muscles also have a postural function through their actions on the ribcage, and she suggests that the rectus abdominis, while a powerful flexor of the lumbar spine, does not play a significant role in respiration. Bunch goes on to state that the main function of the abdominal muscles in respiration is to raise intra-abdominal pressure which in turn aids the upward movement of the relaxed diaphragm by pressing the abdominal viscera onto it.

Subglottic pressure is another factor that must be considered in relation to expiration for singing purposes. '[Subglottic pressure] is a pressure created by the flow of expired air against partially closed (adducted) vocal folds' (Bunch, 1997, p. 51). Subglottic pressure is of some importance to airflow but is vital to achieving a constant intensity of sound. Subglottic pressure is mediated not only by the respiratory system but also by adjustments to the laryngeal musculature.

'In singing, subglottic pressure varies from 2 to 50 cm of H_2O.... To generate a constant subglottic pressure for singing, a graded, co-ordinated action of the inspiratory and expiratory muscles is required, and physiologists, for example Sears (1977), consider the intercostal muscles ideally suited for this task. These muscles have mechanoreceptors which allow fine regulation and gradation in their actions, therefore they are capable of causing delicate adjustments in pressure' (Bunch, 1997, p. 53).

The anatomy and physiology of the respiratory system can seem extremely complex due to the large number of muscles, their interactions and the input of pressure and flow. The most important things to remember are the core concepts we stated at the beginning of the chapter. The respiratory system is all about pressure and flow, balance, flexibility and interaction. The diaphragm is mainly responsible for inhalation, with the team of abdominal muscles (especially the transversus abdominis and the internal and external obliques) mainly responsible for exhalation. The intercostal muscles act for the delicate control of pressure and flow. We can choose to exhale passively or actively by using either elastic recoil or muscular energy!

2

Breathing for singing

There is a continuum in breathing

- breathing for life, tidal breathing (passive exhalation)

- breathing for everyday speech (active exhalation)

- breathing for heightened speech, such as acting, shouting, expletives (active exhalation) and

- breathing for singing (active exhalation).

As we move along the continuum, we need to manage our exhalation more precisely.

Singing is a complex process, requiring lots of interactions amongst the parts that make up the vocal instrument. There is an intimate relationship between the actions of the larynx and the respiratory system. Singing requires not only precise management, but also a component of strength, endurance and flexibility.

While the core concepts regarding breathing for singing appear simple and straightforward, rich folklore has surrounded them, some of which does not match our current scientific understanding.

Information about breathing for singing, some of the science, and some of the methods is detailed below. Of course, if you are already familiar with the core concepts outlined in the box below, you may wish to move on to the next chapter.

Core concepts in breathing for singing

- Singers need to have their breathing under voluntary control.

- Trained singers breathe for speaking in the same way as untrained singers (Hixon and Watson, 1985).

- When singing, trained singers manage their breath differently to untrained singers (Hixon and Watson, 1985).

- Trained singers use greater muscular activity when managing exhalation during singing (Hixon and Watson, 1985).

- Abdominal muscles should be used appropriately to manage exhalation during singing. This muscular activity should remain flexible and dynamic.

- This muscular activity is known as 'support'.

- Support for singing is *not* tension.

- Singers should be able to use supported air flow as required.

- Support should be flexible and dynamic, continuing throughout the phrase.

- Breath management ideally becomes unconscious, driven by the music and text.

- Good postural alignment should be maintained throughout.

- The natural functions and actions of the muscles of inhalation and exhalation should be used.

- Inhalation should be natural and a reflexive action from breathing out.

- 'Overbreathing' ("take as big as a breath as you can") leads to tension. This tension makes it difficult to manage consistent and even airflow.

- The respiratory muscles need strength, flexibility, co-ordination and endurance.

- There are three main schools of breathing for singing related to the position of the abdominal wall:

  - 'Belly in'

  - 'Belly out'

  - Belly neither one nor the other.

- Current research suggests that the 'belly in' school has the most scientific basis.

- Pedagogical writers, such as Vennard, McKinney, White and Chapman, all espouse a form of 'belly in' breath management.

- Accent Method breathing belongs to this 'belly in' school.

- 'When in doubt, breathe out'.

Research into breathing for singing has been somewhat limited compared with the explosion of research into laryngeal mechanics, laryngeal function, acoustics and resonance. Essentially, we can divide the research into two broad types:

- Kinematic investigation

- Electromyography (EMG).

Kinematic studies measure the changes in the dimensions of the chest wall. In kinematic measurement, the chest wall is divided into two parts: the ribcage and the diaphragm/abdomen. Kinematic data can provide information on volume changes, airflow and muscle group activation.

Electromyographic studies aim to identify the presence of electrical activity in a muscle. This activity is a sign that active muscular contraction has taken place. EMGs are particularly useful for identifying which muscles are active at any one time, although EMG responses do not always give accurate information on the *force* of the muscular contraction.

Kinematic studies have given us a significant amount of information about breathing for singing. They are non-invasive; measurements involve the use of belts around the subject's chest and abdomen, or potentiometers positioned to record movement. These measures allow the subject to sing or perform other vocal tasks with little interference.

Early kinematic studies, such as those performed by Watson and Hixon (1987), found that untrained male subjects used respiratory patterns for singing that were very similar to those used for the normal or loud speaking voice. This is consistent with the continuum of breath management; singing (at least in untrained subjects) follows on from the breathing used in loud speaking or shouting. Watson and Hixon were also interested in determining whether there were differences between the trained and the untrained when singing. Initially, only six baritones were studied, but other voice types were used in later research. Watson and Hixon used professional singers who were career soloists.

Overall, Watson and Hixon found that there were very few differences in speaking tasks between the trained and the untrained singers. However, there were significant differences between the trained and untrained singers in singing tasks.

The trained singers showed continuous adjustments to lung volume (i.e., ribcage and abdominal volumes). The changes in lung volumes were also extensive, beginning at quite high volumes and continuing through a large proportion of the vital capacity. Vital capacity refers to how much air is available for use by the lungs. Trained singers used much greater abdominal muscular effort in comparison to untrained singers when singing (Watson and Hixon, 1987, p. 361).

'Overall patterns differed a great deal across subjects, revealing a variety of individual styles of chest wall displacement for singing.' (Watson and Hixon, 1987, p. 361). Interestingly, untrained singers all used very similar patterns of respiratory activity while singing, similar to normal or loud speaking. It appears that instruction or training has a significant effect on the respiratory behaviour of trained singers.

The singer's goal during singing is to ensure that the airflows and pressures generated are efficient for the task at hand. After breathing in, which tends to be deeper for singing than for normal speech, lung volumes are high so the air, which is now under some pressure, is very keen to leave the lungs in a rush. Under these conditions, there is evidence that the inhalatory muscles continue to be active for a significant portion of the exhalation period. They act as releasing brakes, balancing pressure and flow. When the lung volumes fall below a certain point, the exhalatory muscles are solely responsible for continuing to breathe out. These changes appear kinematically as differences in ribcage versus diaphragm/abdomen volumes. Despite individual differences, primarily in timing, research suggests that every trained singer shows gradually smaller and smaller diaphragm/abdominal volumes throughout the sung phrase. There is also some evidence of abdominal activity early in the breathing out cycle.

It is important to remember that Watson and Hixon's statements relate to the activity of the chest wall when the lungs are filled to a high volume. The action of the diaphragm results in the lungs being filled with air, but then to balance the pressures and volumes for a steady stream of air, the ribcage inhalatory muscles are used predominantly, though not exclusively.

Both the inhalatory muscles of the ribcage and the exhalatory muscles of the abdomen are active when the lung volumes are high. This appears to be a contradiction: the exhalatory muscles are actively trying to push air from the body while the inhalatory muscles of the ribcage are actively trying to retain it. Watson and Hixon note that in their trained singers, there was a generalised reduction in abdominal volume, combined with ribcage volume increase. They state that the singer receives an important efficiency gain by activation of the abdomen in these high lung volume circumstances. We know from studies of respiratory physiology that the intercostal muscles are most efficient at high lung volumes. It appears that the abdominal muscles are increasing the pressure on purpose – probably to even up the volumes in the ribcage – to help gain such an advantage.

This seems to suggest that the abdominal muscles are active, performing their exhalatory function regardless of lung volume or inhalatory muscle activity in the ribcage. This finding is important in terms of describing breathing for singing as opposed to breathing for speaking. Therefore, even when there is no obvious need for exhalatory muscle activity, the muscles of the abdominal girdle are recruited for the 'work' of singing.

At mid-lung volume level, most of the exhalatory efforts are abdominal. At low levels, the effort is in both the ribcage and abdomen.

The expiratory efforts of the abdomen serve to displace the diaphragm upwards, which increases the length of the diaphragm's fibres and the radius of its curvature. This mechanically tunes the diaphragm to enable it to function quickly and powerfully as a force generator for inspiration (Watson and Hixon, 1987, p. 364). In addition to the mechanical action on the diaphragm, the abdomen exerts a gentle upward lifting force to the ribcage which naturally elevates it. This action increases its volume and places its expiratory muscles at a greater and more optimal length for quick and forceful pressure changes (Watson and Hixon, 1987, p. 365). Watson and Hixon also point out that the abdominal activity with this group of singers was substantially greater in singing than in speaking. p This confirms the importance of the abdominal wall in breathing for singing.

For Watson and Hixon, the most prevalent style of inspiration seemed to involve both ribcage and abdominal volume increases. In some subjects there was a simultaneous, symmetrical change in both ribcage and abdominal wall volumes. In others there was an abdominal volume increase followed by a ribcage volume increase.

The singer's goal during inhalation is to breathe in quickly and efficiently. Watson and Hixon state that the diaphragm is primarily responsible for the in-breath while the abdominal muscles relax. The diaphragm can be identified as the prime mover in inhalation due to the large outward movements of the abdomen. This is supported by the work of Bouhuys and colleagues (1966) and Proctor (1968, reported in Proctor, 1980) which demonstrated high transdiaphragmatic pressure in singers during inhalation. This is consistent with vigorous diaphragm contraction.

The diaphragm is the most powerful of all the inhalatory muscles and, through its action, displaces both the ribcage and the abdomen. The use of the diaphragm for the in-breath then leaves the ribcage free of inspiratory work. The ribcage can then begin to manage pressure and flow during expiration. The diaphragm can be continuously tuned mechanically by the abdomen, as mentioned above, regardless of lung volume, to work as quickly and as efficiently as possible for the next in-breath (Watson and Hixon, 1987, p. 366).

Watson and Hixon made some interesting observations on the transition between breathing in and breathing out. The main transition involved activation of the abdominal muscles to help pressurise the chest with air.

The transition between breathing out and breathing in is also an important part of the respiratory cycle for singing.

When viewing kinematic data the exhalation to inhalation transition appears to show a reduction in ribcage volume but a relatively large increase in abdominal volume. This is most likely due to the action of the diaphragm, which opens the lower ribs and displaces the abdominal contents down and slightly forward. At the same time the sternum will fall slightly as the diaphragm opens the ribcage from below. In many singers some increase in ribcage volume may then follow.

It is possible to summarise the results of these kinematic studies more simply. There is co-ordinated and organised activity in the diaphragm, ribcage wall and abdominal musculature throughout the breathing cycle in trained singers. It appears as though the diaphragm is primarily responsible for inhalation with the abdominal muscles active during expiration in a role that assists the pressurisation of the chest with air, so that the ribcage can more easily control pressure and flow.

In their 1985 experiments, Watson and Hixon used only male singers. A similar study using female singers was carried out by Watson, Hixon, Stathopoulos and Sullivan in 1990. There were no significant differences between the male and female singers.

Proctor, in his 1980 book *Breathing, speech and song*, reports on some early experiments which evaluated ribcage and abdominal activity during singing, undertaken on himself as subject. Proctor was not only a Professor of Otolaryngology and a respiratory researcher, but also a highly trained professional singer. His conclusions regarding breathing for singing are remarkably similar to those drawn by Watson and Hixon. He believes that the diaphragm is mainly involved in inhalation, the intercostal muscles control the pressure and airflow for much of the exhalation, and the abdominal wall moves inward to assist in the control of the outward flow of air.

Thorpe *et al.* (2001) studied the difference between fully supported and less well supported singing in a group of five professional singers. They recruited singers who had been trained by a single teacher and so, presumably, followed a consistent method of breathing and support. Although this study focuses primarily on the differences between supported and less well supported singing, the kinematic data obtained is of interest.

Chapman (one of the authors) was the singing teacher who trained all the subjects used in this study. She teaches a method which '... emphasises the use of abdominal support synchronised with the onset of phonation' (Thorpe *et al.*, 2001, p. 87). Chapman believes that the main muscles used for this abdominal support are the transverse abdominis and the internal and external obliques. As part of the process of learning her method of breathing and support she uses primal sounds such as cries, sobs, laughs and yells. Such sounds appear to evoke actions in the muscles mentioned naturally.

'Chapman teaches that all singing should be supported [with these muscles], but it is noticeable that during 'projected singing there is a particular increase in muscle contraction in the lateral abdominal region. This lateral abdominal support appears to provide stability to the actions of the ribcage and diaphragm during phonation' (Thorpe *et al.*, 2001, p. 87).

Chapman also insists that this support is not active during inhalation and she asks the singer to release abdominal tension at the start of inspiration so that the diaphragm can descend quickly. She terms this onomatopoeically 'SPLAT'. Dinah Harris, one of her colleagues, has since turned SPLAT into the following mnemonic: 'Singers Please Loosen Abdominal Tension' (Chapman, 2006, p. 41).

Thorpe *et al.* indicate that although there are some minor differences in the recordings due to the subjects singing different repertoire, there are notable similarities between subjects' respiratory patterns. Inhalation commences with a rapid manoeuvre in which there is expansion in the abdomen occurring concurrently with a decrease in ribcage volume. This manoeuvre results in a negligible volume change and is very short – in the order of only 100 milliseconds (Thorpe *et al.*, 2001, p. 90). After this, inhalation continues with expansion in both the ribcage and the abdomen. This is followed by a further realignment consisting of a simultaneous elevation of the ribcage and a drawing in of the abdomen. Vocalisation usually commences part way through this alignment. Exhalation continues with a simultaneous decrease in both ribcage and abdominal dimensions (Thorpe *et al.*, 2001, pp. 90–92).

Thorpe *et al.* note that the ribcage volume changes in the ribcage and abdominal wall correspond well with the pedagogical instruction given to the singers. They also note that the paradoxical ribcage–abdomen movement described at the start of inspiration is consistent with the data generated by Watson and Hixon (1985) and described again in Hixon's 1987 book. Although Watson and Hixon reported a wider variety of respiratory patterns, the most experienced singers in their study were reported to have ribcage and abdominal volume patterns that were very similar to those shown by the subjects in the Thorpe *et al* study.

Thorpe *et al.* also note that in conditions of increased support, there is an increase in the lateral dimensions of the ribcage coupled with a decrease in abdominal volume. 'The dimension changes are suggestive of an increased abdominal pressure with the greater 'support' evoked for the projected condition' (2001, p. 102). They also postulate that 'simultaneous activation of the ribcage and abdominal muscles may result in more rapid and possibly better controlled changes in subglottal pressure' (Thorpe *et al.*, 2001, p. 102).

In conclusion, Thorpe *et al.* believe that 'the use of support exhibits itself … as a movement away from the relaxation state, with abdominal muscle activation and the raising of the ribcage, coupled with a rapid release of expiratory muscle activity at the start of inspiration' (2001, p. 103).

The consistency of the data in the Thorpe *et al.* study (2001) suggests that the training offered to singers and the concepts taught about breathing can significantly affect the respiratory choices made by them in performance. The pedagogy used in this study follows the natural function of respiratory physiology. Inhalation is essentially under the control of the diaphragm. During exhalation there is active participation of the abdominal muscles to increase abdominal pressure and tune the diaphragm for the next inhalation. The pressures required for phonation appear to be under the control of the ribcage.

A common thread running through the research into breathing for singing is that although some common or generalised conclusions can be drawn from the scientific data, there is a degree of variability in the singer's methods. Control of the subglottic pressure is the prime focus of the breathing apparatus during phonation for singing. Despite the fact that some singers appear to have an idiosyncratic method of achieving it, they all do so to a rather high degree of proficiency.

Hixon continued his researches into the respiratory function for singing until his death in 2009. His 2006 publication, *Respiratory function in singing: A primer for singers and singing teachers*, summarises his work and confirms the statements made in his earlier research. A number of important concepts are stressed in his book, particularly the role of the ribcage and abdominal wall in singing:

'The ribcage wall and abdominal wall are active during most continuous singing phrases. ... Both the ribcage wall and abdominal wall squeeze during continuous singing phrases but the squeeze of the abdominal wall is more forceful than that of the ribcage wall'. (Hixon, 2006, p. 97) [We are quoting directly here; 'squeeze' would not be our choice of word!].

'Thus, the preferred muscular strategy for continuous singing increases the efficiency of chest wall function. By forcefully and continuously activating the abdominal wall, the background shape of the chest wall is mechanically tuned to favour the inspiratory function of the diaphragm and expiratory function of the ribcage wall'. (Hixon, 2006, p. 99).

Hixon has made it clear that the abdominal wall is vitally important in singing. Based on the work of Thorpe *et al.* (2001), it would also appear that the abdominal wall is vital to the notion of 'support' in classical singing.

EMG studies have been used to evaluate the respiratory system for singers. Leanderson and Sundberg reported on needle EMG findings from the diaphragm in their summary article on breathing for singing, published in *Journal of Voice* in 1988. They found that the four singers studied showed two different patterns of diaphragm activity: the diaphragm was either continuously contracting throughout the phrase, or it was entirely inactive throughout the phrase, activating for inhalation only (Leanderson and Sundberg, 1988, p. 4).

Watson *et al.* (1989) used surface EMG to evaluate the activity of the abdominal muscles during singing. They used four male singers, all professionals, who had undergone at least 10 years of singing training. EMG was recorded from four sites on the abdomen: upper and lower lateral, and upper and lower middle. Kinematic data were recorded at the same time (Watson *et al.*, 1989, p. 25). In addition to a number of respiratory manoeuvres, singers were recorded speaking and reading, as well as singing two stylistically contrasting Italian songs: *Amarilli mia Bella*, by Caccini, and *Che Fiero Costume*, by Legrenzi. These two songs were also used by Watson and Hixon in their 1985 kinematic study.

Watson *et al.* found that there was almost no observable activity in the mid-line sites during tidal breathing. Some activity was noted at the lateral sites, with more activity recorded at the lower than the upper site (1989, p. 26). During speaking tasks, there was clearly observable activity at the lateral sites, combined with slight or no observable activity in the middle sites. For three of the four subjects, there was more activity in the lower lateral than upper lateral sites (Watson *et al.*, 1989, p. 27). 'This pattern is suggestive of activation of the external oblique abdominis, internal oblique abdominis, transverse abdominis, or some combination of these muscles, with little or no activation of the rectus abdominis' (Watson *et al.*, 1989, p. 28). Watson *et al.* (1989) also indicated that this pattern of results was not significantly different from the results obtained from a group. of subjects without professional training or experience. The EMG data are in agreement with the kinematic data in suggesting that there are no significant differences between trained singers and untrained speakers on speaking tasks.

During singing there was a substantial increase in the EMG activity of the abdomen. Once again there was more activity recorded at the lower lateral site than at the upper lateral site, and there was substantially more activity in the lateral sites than in the mid-line sites (Watson *et al.*, 1989, p. 28). Subjects demonstrated high amplitude EMG activity in both middle and lateral regions during the production of a loud, sustained, high-pitched note, such as that which occurred at the end of *Che Fiero Costume*, by Legrenzi (Watson *et al.*, 1989, p. 28). Once again, kinematic data were in agreement with the EMG traces, and were very similar to those obtained by Watson and Hixon in their 1895 study. During exhalation, the results can be summarised as follows:

'The lowest overall levels of activation were associated with relaxing and the highest with singing. For breathing, speaking and singing, abdominal activity was greater in the lateral region than the middle region. Differential activation within the lateral region was observed with activity in the lower portion exceeding that of the upper portion'. (Watson *et al.*, 1989, p. 29)

It is important to note that EMG activity in the abdominal wall was quite specific, which renders dubious the findings of other studies that have relied on single electrode site recordings. Absence of EMG activity from a single site on the abdomen cannot be equated with absence of activity of the abdominal wall as a whole (Watson *et al.*, 1989, p. 30).

During inhalation, there was a decrease in the EMG activity of the abdominal wall associated with the in-breath. 'Such decrements began either coincident with, or slightly prior to the onset of inspiration and were present in both lateral sites, or in the lower lateral site only' (Watson *et al.*, 1989, p. 30). When the kinematic data were also analysed, it became obvious that 'for both speaking and singing, decrements often were associated with outward displacement of the abdomen.' (Watson *et al.*, 1989, p. 30). The decreases showed activity that was often as minimal as that recorded in the relaxation manoeuvres. It is thought that the decreases in abdominal activity associated with the in-breath reduce the resistance of the abdomen to the descending diaphragm. This allows diaphragmatic contraction to be seen as outward abdominal wall displacement. This lack of resistance to the descending diaphragm would allow a more efficient and effective in-breath (Watson *et al.*, 1989, p. 30). These decreases were brief in duration and there was a natural rapid return of abdominal activity before the inhalation was completed.

In conclusion, abdominal activity is clearly present during singing, with the lateral sites more active than the medial ones. Deactivation of the abdominal wall is seen on inhalation, and this appears to assist the mechanical action of the diaphragm. However, the abdominal wall reactivates quickly to resume its role of posturing the entire chest wall for singing (Watson *et al.*, 1989, p. 31).

Sundberg *et al.* (1991) also carried out EMG studies of the respiratory muscles used in singing. They remind us that singers have finely tuned control over the subglottal pressures produced while singing. Subglottal pressure controls vocal loudness as well as exerting an influence on the pitch (p. 283). '… singers have to tailor subglottal pressure individually for each note, taking into account both its loudness and pitch. As subglottal pressure affects the fundamental frequency, the intended target pressures must be matched quite accurately for the singer to stay on pitch' (Sundberg *et al.*, 1991, p. 283–284).

Sundberg *et al.* (1991) took EMG recordings from the internal and external intercostals, the diaphragm, and from the abdominal oblique muscle. The singers involved were asked to perform a number of vocal tasks but sang neither an aria nor song.

The results of this study were quite similar to those obtained by Watson *et al.* (1989), and confirm that the abdominal wall is actively engaged in configuring the chest wall during singing. Relaxation, or at least inhibition of its activity, also occurs during inhalation. The diaphragm is active during inhalation and there is activity in the intercostal muscles throughout much of the breath cycle.

Given these findings concerning breathing for singing gleaned from the scientific literature it is possible to draw some conclusions about an appropriate method of breathing for singing. When exhalation is active and the intra-abdominal pressure assists in the control of the outward flow of air, some interaction of the inhalatory and exhalatory muscles is required. It appears that this interaction of the muscles forms the basis of breath support. As the muscles of respiration are mostly striated muscles and thus, under voluntary control, systematic training should enable the singer to develop fine breath control. We believe that an effective breath support system for singing therefore consists of:

- Voluntary control of respiratory muscles, allowing the singer to increase or decrease support and breath flow at will

- Efficient, flexible use of the respiratory physiology

- Freedom from tension in the upper chest and neck

- Maintenance of good postural alignment

- A system of breath management that follows the natural functions of the inhalatory and exhalatory muscles

- Training of the respiratory muscles in terms of strength, co-ordination and endurance.

Breathing and breath management in the vocal pedagogical literature

There is perhaps no part of vocal pedagogy that has been so hotly contested over the years as breathing. Many different schools of breathing have developed, each claiming to be the one true and correct method. These schools of breathing can be broadly divided into three. Those that expound a 'belly in' method of supporting the voice, those that are completely opposite in approach and propose a 'belly out' method of support and, finally, those pedagogues who choose neither. There are differences in exact technique amongst the different adherents to each school, but the direction of movement of the abdomen (the prime mover in expiration) remains the same for all.

Almost all pedagogues believe that breathing, breath support, or breath management is part of a solid vocal technique. The degree to which breathing is felt to be important varies greatly from one pedagogue to another.

The growth of scientific knowledge about the respiratory system has tended to marginalise the 'belly out' school in more recent times, particularly as kinematic studies, such as those reported by Hixon in his 1987 book, make it clear that inward movement of the abdomen was recorded in all singers during the expiration phase, regardless of how they conceptualised their breathing for singing (p. 362). While very little has been written in the last 20 to 30 years to suggest the use of the 'belly out' strategy for singing, it is still taught by some teachers despite all the scientific developments in respiration that are now available in the literature. Interestingly, other than for voice, the 'belly out' method of breath support is still a common method of breathing among wind instrumentalists, and references to its use are often found in wind and brass pedagogies (Reynolds, 2005).

McKinney points out that all methods of breathing, be they correct or incorrect, usually have some element of truth in them. Students who are taught belly breathing are instructed to 'take a deep breath and then push out against your belt while you sing. This has the effect of locking the diaphragm in the lowest position to which it has descended and not allowing it to make its return as air is expended' (McKinney, 1994, p. 60). It is true that the diaphragm must be allowed to descend as fully as is possible, the element of truth in the belly breathing school, but the diaphragm must also be allowed to return to its un-contracted state during the breath cycle. The abdominal muscles must also remain free to move inward in order to maintain the balance of air pressure required for singing. The 'belly out' theory has been essentially laid to waste by the research findings from respiratory kinematics. The 'belly in' and 'neither one nor the other' schools of breathing can be assessed by examining some of the other writings on vocal pedagogy.

Many of today's pedagogues base their beliefs about breathing and breath management for singing on the writings or teachings from the so called 'Golden Age' of Bel Canto singing. It is important to remember that pedagogues in historical times had no access to scientific tools for investigating how their breathing systems worked and relied solely on their own sensations as singers, and on the information available to them from the anatomy laboratory. We know that the singer's own perception of how the breath management or breath support system works often bears little resemblance to what actually happens physiologically (Watson and Hixon, 1987, p. 370). Anatomy laboratories are excellent places to observe structures and to trace the origins and insertions of muscles but, due to the complex interactions that occur between muscles (in particular) in live subjects, it is often difficult to give accurate descriptions of the functions of the muscles themselves, or to give clear and precise descriptions of how systems such as the entire respiratory system work. We now have a much better understanding of muscular actions, and the interactions amongst structures within a system, thanks to tools such as electromyography, X-ray, ultrasound, manometry and kinematics.

A brief overview of some of the earlier writings is valuable, as these authors may have influenced the work of more modern pedagogues; to some extent they may also have driven the way in which scientific research has been assimilated into current pedagogy.

Some of the earliest writings on singing, those of Tosi and Mancini, have nothing specific to say about breathing. It is the castrati, the keepers of vocal knowledge from the first Bel Canto era, who were reputed to have the secrets of vocal pedagogy, including breathing. As only limited numbers of technical exercises were written down and described, much of what they taught has been lost. The Garcias (the elder and the younger) were perhaps the first to write in some detail about the technical aspects of singing. Garcia (the elder) exhorted students to breathe slowly and without noise but his son, Garcia the younger, whose pedagogy was built upon that of his father, used specific breathing exercises to give power and elasticity to the lungs. There remains a common misconception that the lungs have a role to play in breath management. We now know that the lungs are basically air-filled sacs, and that breath is managed by muscles in the thorax and diaphragm.

Garcia (the younger) did, however, recognise the interaction between breathing and posture. 'Shoulders thrown back without stiffness and the chest expanded, the diaphragm lowered without any jerk, and the chest regularly and slowly raised' (Coffin, 1989, p. 32). Garcia termed complete inhalation 'respiro', with the half breath or 'mezzo-respiro' also taught. Garcia correctly allots the prime place for inhalation as the diaphragm, and he also correctly identifies posture as important when breathing for singing. He also makes much of the in-breath in his exercises, such as 'inhalation very slowly through pursed lips until the chest is full, and the lungs filled then the breath is held for as long as possible' (Coffin, 1989, p. 33),and suggested the slow expiration of air from a deep breath. It appears that these exercises were carried out separately from singing.

The Garcias appear to have been among the first to use the term 'diaphragmatic breathing', since it is credited to them by a number of later writers. Today we also recognise the term 'diaphragmatic breathing', despite differences in the perception of the term. Many of the older sources appear to credit the diaphragm with an expiratory function that simply does not exist. In more modern times, diaphragmatic breathing refers to the descent of the diaphragm during the in-breath, which is usually coupled with abdominal control of the out-breath. This is consistent with the physiological fact that the diaphragm is a muscle of inspiration only. Some of the more modern pedagogies still exhort students to 'sing from the diaphragm', but this appears to be an image that has existed almost from the beginning of vocal pedagogy, despite having no real basis in physiological fact (Watson and Hixon, 1987, p 370).

Matilda Marchesi, another famous pedagogue who was Dame Nellie Melba's teacher, insisted on normal breathing in which the lungs are expanded at the base to give the greatest quantity of air. She also believed that posture was important to breath. Marchesi made comments about the use of corsetry, which restricted abdominal movement, firmly believing that tight corsets caused 'lateral breathing' which was detrimental. Without the benefit of modern scientific equipment, she appears to have correctly identified a number of necessary physiological facts. The concept of the lungs expanding at the base can be seen to relate to the descent of the diaphragm, while her abhorrence of corsetry which restricted abdominal distension indicates that she understood the relationship between the descent of the diaphragm and the movement of the viscera downwards and outwards.

Other pedagogues, teaching at a similar time to Marchesi, did not agree with her, particularly in relation to the concept of a 'normal breath'. Stockhausen, for example, felt that diaphragmatic breathing was sufficient for the mezzo respiro, but that extension of the ribs for the respiro pieno (deep or full breath) was indispensable. Stockhausen seemed to believe that the ribs and the diaphragm worked completely independently of each other, a belief that we now know to be, in the main, erroneous.

The Lampertis - Father, Francesco and son, Giovanni Battista - have probably had the greatest influence on breathing for singing: they were the first to coin the terms 'appoggio' and the 'lutte vocale' (vocal struggle). The appoggio is first mentioned in Francesco Lamperti's 1890 book: 'The appoggio, or support of the voice, was to be gained by the action of the muscles of the chest and diaphragm upon the lungs after opening the lower part of the throat on the vowel 'a' [X-ray photography indicates this is a vocal imagery]' (Coffin, 1989, p. 59). In some ways, Lamperti is correct in that the lungs are acted upon by muscles which are not directly attached to them, but he is also ascribing to the diaphragm an expiratory function that modern science has proved it simply does not have. From this description of appoggio, direct from Lamperti, it is clear that the concept of appoggio in this form is not based on physiological fact.

In common with other earlier pedagogues, Francesco Lamperti tends to focus on the in-breath, with an instruction to singers to direct their attentions to the full inhalation of up to 18 seconds (similar to the Garcias). Despite making erroneous statements about the diaphragm's expiratory function, Lamperti makes a number of correct statements, such as those in his description of the lutte vocale: 'With the full breath the diaphragm is lowered pressing on the organs below. When singing occurred, the inspiratory muscles struggled against the expiratory muscles to retain breath within the body. This he called the lutte vocale, or 'vocal struggle" ...' (Coffin, 1989, p. 61). We now know from kinematic studies such as those of Watson and Hixon (1985) that this vocal struggle does in fact exist. When the lungs are full of air, the elastic recoil of the system is attempting to expel the excess air from the lungs, while inspiratory muscles in the ribcage and the diaphragm continue to function to maintain an appropriate thoracic pressure. At the same time, the abdominal wall is also acting (expiratory function) to tune and posture both the diaphragm and the rest of the chest wall. Our current understanding is that the action of the abdominal wall raises the intra-abdominal pressure which in turn raises the intra-thoracic pressure. This increased intra-thoracic pressure triggers the mechano-pressure receptors that are within the ribcage wall, encouraging ongoing action of the diaphragm and intercostal muscles during the breath cycle. The mechanical push of the abdominal contents upwards onto the diaphragm also has the effect of altering its posture and stretching its fibres, tuning it for the next descent on the in-breath.

Francesco's son, Giovanni Battista, also made some correct statements about breathing. He believed that the manner of breathing should be diaphragmatic, as this was the only method that allowed singers to control the air with tranquillity. He also noted that strain was placed on the voice by the use of high or clavicular breathing, and that posture and breath interacted. Giovanni Battista believed that the control of the breath was the foundation of all vocal study. He also appeared to be slightly more accurate in his description of the out-breath when he stated: 'Expiration should be effected chiefly by the abdominal muscles in a gradual manner to spin out the tone' (Coffin, 1989, p. 64).

Giovanni Battista Lamperti's student and assistant teacher, William Earl Brown, wrote the book *Vocal Wisdom* in the 1930s (revised and expanded in the 1950s), based on the maxims of Lamperti that he heard firsthand as a student and then as assistant teacher. It is interesting to note the use of imagery, much of which is not based on physiological fact, which was used for teaching. It is also possible to see how myths and traditions could be passed down as fact, rather than as teaching images. The paragraphs in Brown's book on incorporated breath are an excellent example of this.

'The whole torso contracts and expands co-ordinately. The shoulders and hips are linked together to prevent expansion while filling the lungs for the purpose of singing. The pelvic region and breast bone mutually bear the strain of the energy of the inspired air. The force of this compressed breath crowds upward toward the 'wish bone' causing the singer to feel broad shouldered and high chested. (The breast bone is attached to each shoulder)....Then the voice begins to vibrate, the diaphragm permits enough breath energy to escape to produce and feed the pulsations that we call tone – and without push or pull of muscle'. (Brown, 1957, p. 108).

Lamperti, through Brown, or rather Brown's interpretation of what Lamperti told him, is correct physiologically in the following ways: the torso does work as a unit in a coordinated fashion to manage breath; both the pelvic area and the breast bone (sternum) have muscular attachments that can be easily palpated during supported phonation (laughing, crying, sobbing and correct singing); and the singer should feel broad shouldered, upright and 'noble' (though because of posture not the breath itself). This passage, unfortunately, also contains a number of quite erroneous statements. If there is no expansion of the epigastric area as the diaphragm descends, the breathing will be high and somewhat limited in amount, so if the shoulders and hips are linked to prevent expansion it would be very difficult for the lungs to fill with air. The diaphragm is again ascribed an expiratory function: it does not control the outward flow of air. It may act as a brake to the expiratory force of the abdominal muscles, but it certainly does not control overall expiratory energy. Finally, the statements that muscles are not involved, neither push, nor pull, must certainly be an image. Inspiratory muscles must continue to work, initially to overcome the elastic recoil of the system just after the inhalation, or much of the breath would be lost too quickly. Then, once the intra-thoracic pressure has dropped sufficiently, expiratory muscles must come into play to take over the control of the outward flow of air.

Throughout much of the early part of the twentieth century, these types of pedagogical statements were used and passed to students as fact, rather than as images. During the 1950s, there was a great deal of interest from anatomists, physiologists and voice researchers into how the breath was used to sustain life and for the purposes of speaking. Pedagogues began to be influenced by this research, and the work of William Vennard is a prime example of this early interaction between singing pedagogues and scientists.

Vennard's 1967 book, *Singing: The mechanism and the technic*, was a cornerstone of pedagogical literature for most of the latter part of the twentieth century. Vennard described his book as frankly mechanistic, and he attempted to demystify singing and couch it in purely scientific terms '[this book] is an attempt to compile under one cover objective findings from various reliable sources and relate them to the art of singing' (Vennard, 1967, p. iii).

Vennard believed that breathing was central to an efficient vocal technique.

> 'There are those teachers who consider breathing the most important factor in tone production....Conversely, poor singing is directly the result of poor breathing, that consequently there is a just one thing to teach in the studio – correct inhalation and exhalation'. (Vennard, 1967, p. 18).

Vennard also stated that 'it [breathing] is primary in importance, but it is easy to understand and can be practised without the aid of a teacher' (Vennard, 1967, p. 18). Vennard's basis for stating this was that all the muscles involved in respiration can be voluntarily controlled. Certainly, this appears to be true to some extent. Even the diaphragm can be activated to initiate a breath by conscious thought, even if the fine graduation of its movement may not be under our voluntary control.

From his position in the middle of the twentieth century, Vennard was able to draw conclusions from some of the other singing pedagogies, either by direct interaction with some of their chief practitioners, or with singers who had been taught themselves by the founders of these pedagogies. He notes that there are quite a few singers who are successful, in spite of what appear to be poor breathing habits, especially mentioning Lilli Lehman. Lilli Lehman was one of the great sopranos of the early twentieth century who for most of her career championed 'pan-costal' breathing. Pan-costal breathing required that the abdomen be drawn tightly in on the in-breath, so that the chest could fill with air (not physiologically sound at all!). It was only later in her career that Lehman learned to release the abdominal wall to allow the diaphragm a quick and easy descent. Vennard rightly points out that everyone does breathe and as long as the air goes in and flows out again with reasonable steadiness, singing can occur. However, he also states that if the breath can be increased, so, too, can the quality of the singing. (Vennard, 1967, p. 18).

Vennard also makes a strong connection between good posture and good breathing, and he likens the posture of the singer to the task that instrumentalists face when learning to hold their instruments correctly before beginning to play.

> 'The head, chest and pelvis should be supported by the spine in such a way that they will align themselves one under the other – head erect, chest high, pelvis tipped so that the tail is tucked in. The position of the head and shoulders allows the jaw to be free, not pulled back into the throat. This 3liberates the organs in the neck. The high chest implies that the shoulders go back, but they should relax and feel comfortable….A certain amount of tonicity of the abdominal muscles will be needed to keep the pelvis upright, but there must not be so much that deep breathing is impossible. This aspect of posture should be ignored if it prevents abdominal breathing' (Vennard, 1967, p. 19).

Vennard correctly identifies the need for the abdominal muscles to relax, to allow the diaphragm a quick and easy descent. In many ways, well before the term was coined, Vennard was asking the singer to maintain core stability, but allow freedom in the abdominal wall to assist breathing for singing. Vennard also stated that 'There must also be an expansion of the ribs to provide leverage for the muscles of breathing' (Vennard, 1967, p. 20). It appears that he believes that the ribs can move independently of structures such as the diaphragm, although Rubin (1998) and Bunch

(1997) make it clear that the lower ribs, in particular, move because of the diaphragm's attachment to them, rather than separate from it.

'Respiration is a complex physiological process of which phonation is only a secondary function. For purposes of study it may be analysed into three types of breathing: chest, rib and diaphragmatic or abdominal. The first should be de-emphasised; the most efficient breathing for singing is a combination of the latter two'. (Vennard, 1967, p. 20).

Vennard has again made a correct statement when he identifies the combination of rib-diaphragmatic and abdominal breathing as the most efficient for singing. These two types of breathing equate to the actions of the primary inspiratory and expiratory muscles, as described by Hixon (1987), while his descriptions of 'chest' breathing relate most closely to the actions of the secondary muscles of inspiration. Vennard is perhaps one of the first singing pedagogues to use accurate anatomical and physiological information to support his breathing pedagogy. Because of his understanding of correct anatomy and physiology, he is firmly within the 'belly in' school of breathing.

Vennard's description of the respiratory system is essentially correct, although he does ascribe to the older anatomists' descriptions of the functions of the internal and external intercostal muscles, with one group responsible for inhalation and the other for exhalation. Rubin (1998) and Bunch (1997) state that the intercostals act to stabilise the ribcage wall and to assist in maintaining correct intra-thoracic pressure, rather than being responsible for the increase and decrease of lung volumes. In his desire to be anatomically accurate, Vennard does mention the fact that the fibres of the intercostal muscles do change their direction of pull as their attachments get closer to the sternum, which would of course change their function, if it were truly to control lung volumes. Vennard's statements about the diaphragm are also completely accurate, and he even comments on the close interaction between the ribs and the diaphragm, although he does not appear to understand that it is the diaphragm's movement rather than the movement of the ribs that predominates in the inspiratory cycle. 'Naturally, this flattening of the dome (of the diaphragm) will be co-ordinated with the expanding of the ribs, to which it is attached at its circumference' (Vennard, 1967, p. 24). Vennard also made use of radiographic studies to back up his statements. X-ray studies prove that the diaphragm always descends on inhalation and it descends radically on deep breathing (Vennard, 1967, p. 24).

Vennard makes comments about the muscles of the abdomen and pelvic floor, which he believes are vital for good breathing for singing:

> 'Needless to say, the action of these muscles [pelvic floor] is instinctive, as is the case with most of the respiratory musculature. Training these muscles consists of conditioning these reflexes into patterns which are more efficient for singing and this only modifies the overall behaviour somewhat.' (Vennard, 1967, p. 25)

In making such statements about the 'instinctive' or 'reflexive' nature of these muscular movements, Vennard is alluding to a vital component of any vocal technique: that it must be physiologically appropriate. It is not sound practice to ask a singer to move muscles or use muscular systems in ways for which the body is not designed. The most efficient use must be made of physiology and this will usually occur when the body is allowed to make its own choices about how it will function.

Chest breathing, which is also known as clavicular or shoulder breathing, is described by Vennard as the breathing of the exhausted athlete or the person who is out of breath and gasping for air. The heaving chest that is associated with this type of breathing is a sign that the body is struggling to get enough oxygen for life. Vennard advises against this type of breathing for four reasons:

> 'First, it is inefficient. It is inspiratory and provides no control over exhalation….Second, it looks bad. When a singer collapses his chest, his shoulders droop and his posture becomes poor….Third, chest breathing can easily lead to muscular tension in the throat. The muscles that raise the breast bone have attachments at the top of the

neck....Fourth, abdominal breathing which is best cannot take place correctly when the ribs are heaving.' (Vennard, 1967, p. 27).

The second type of respiration is characterised by the sideways expansion of the ribs which Vennard terms costal or rib breathing. With the heels of the hands placed against the lower ribs at the sides and the fingers lightly touching in front: 'When he [the singer] inhales, his objective will be to push them [the hands] as far apart as possible' (Vennard, 1967, p. 28). Vennard also points out that some great teachers, such as Marchesi, did not believe in costal breathing any more than in clavicular breathing. 'They felt that the rib muscles should only be used to expand the ribs and keep them in this position, making possible the most efficient operation of lower muscles, the true motors of breathing' (Vennard 1967, p. 28). Vennard goes on to point out that 'the normal expansion of the ribs is primarily sidewards, partly forward and very little upward so that it co-ordinates with belly rather than shoulder breathing' (Vennard, 1967, p. 28).

Vennard appears to understand the link between the lower ribs and the diaphragm, since he indicates that the rib movements co-ordinate with the abdominals rather than the shoulders. However, he is in error as he feels that the ribs could have quite independent movement from the diaphragm. More recent writers (Bunch, 1997 and Rubin, 1998) believe that the diaphragm is the prime mover of the lower ribs, with the intercostal muscles mainly concerned with maintaining ribcage integrity and preventing the ribcage from being sucked in by the negative pressure in the thorax created by the descending diaphragm. The attachment of the diaphragm to the lower ribs also ensures that they swing outwards (Vennard's sideways movement) on inspiration.

The third type of breathing described by Vennard is diaphragmatic-abdominal or 'belly- breathing'. It is, in essence, diaphragmatic during inhalation and abdominal during exhalation.

'The diaphragm is one of the most powerful muscles in the body, and certainly a most important one. It is not only a partition between the ribcage and the belly, but it is related to both types of breathing and thus implies that they should be co-ordinated'. (Vennard, 1967, p. 28).

Vennard goes on to give an excellent explanation of how the diaphragm moves and how its movement impinges on the abdominal contents. He also comments on how the bulge at the level of the epigastrium relates indirectly to diaphragm movement. 'When it [the diaphragm] flattens, this area will push forward. Plunket Greene [a famous baritone of the early twentieth century] called it the 'breathing muscle' (Vennard, 1967, p. 28). It is, of course, not the diaphragm at all, something that many pedagogues have quoted erroneously for years, but the sensation of the movement of some of the stomach contents and other muscle junctions, caused by the descent of the diaphragm.

Vennard reiterates that a combination of rib and belly breathing is the best possible technique.

'The contraction of the diaphragm causes it to lower and partly flatten, increasing the capacity of the thorax. It is the muscle of inhalation. The contraction of the abdominal muscles decreases the capacity of the entire trunk, including the thorax except in certain functions. They are the muscles of exhalation. They are resisted and steadied in their contraction by the diaphragm, but it only causes confusion to think of this muscle being the active factor. The diaphragm does not support the tone....The diaphragm steadies the tone but does not support it..' (Vennard, 1967, p. 30).

Vennard is making a clear statement about physiological fact, with which he aims to debunk the long held view that the diaphragm somehow manages to contract for inhalation, and then relax in such a way that it actively supports the air on exhalation and controls the voice. Vennard's belief that the diaphragm steadies the tone has not been conclusively proven, but in a study by Sundberg and his coworkers, it was found that singers usually recruited the diaphragm to rapidly decrease subglottic pressure at high lung volumes (Sundberg, 1987, p.

IF IN DOUBT, BREATHE OUT!

36). Sundberg's experimental group was very small, only four subjects, and no mention was made as to their level of skill. One of his subjects showed diaphragmatic activity throughout the duration of the sung phrase. Sundberg also reported that this singer tended to generate a higher subglottic pressure with his abdominal wall, which was then reduced to the required pressure by the activity of the diaphragm. Sundberg postulates that this high degree of concomitant contraction helps reduce the displacement of the abdominal contents and thus, minimises the influence of their inertia on a rapidly changing subglottic pressure.

This analogy of the accelerator and the brake, with the abdominal wall being the accelerator and the diaphragm the brake, would explain the results that Sundberg obtained. Interestingly, this accelerator/brake concept is core to the pedagogical model of breathing taught by Janice Chapman and expounded in her book, *Singing and teaching singing: A holistic approach to classical voice* (2006).

Sundberg also cites other earlier papers, such as Bouhuys *et al.* (1966) who found that three out of five non-professional singers used the diaphragm to reduce the respiratory recoil forces for singing long, soft, sustained tones at high lung volumes (Sundberg, 1987, p. 37).

Vennard also attempts to explain the phenomenon of the 'bouncing epigastrium' which many pedagogues have used as a proof of good diaphragmatic development. He rightly points out that the bulging of the epigastrium occurs due to muscular interactions between the diaphragm and the abdominal muscles, not from the diaphragm alone. Vennard correctly identifies this 'bouncing' as a result of reflexive muscular interactions, since it occurs quite clearly in coughing (as well as in other primal or primitive noises such as laughter, sobbing or crying). He also makes it clear that the abdominal muscles are responsible for the rapid expulsion of air caused during coughing, although he does make note of the fact that the diaphragm will also tense to help control the force of the outgoing air stream (Vennard, 1967, p. 31).

Vennard appears to deserve his place as one of the 'greats' of vocal pedagogy of the twentieth century. He critically examined the language and practices of vocal pedagogues and attempted to relate them to the scientific principles of his day. Apart from a few minor additions to our knowledge, such as information about the intercostal muscles gained through electromyographical and kinematic studies, Vennard's descriptions of respiratory anatomy and physiology are correct. He has usually interpreted the language and practices of the pedagogue correctly and has made clear and concise scientific connections. Vennard's claim that a combination of rib and belly breathing (we now call this abdomino-diaphragmatic breathing) is the best for singing fits well with current physiological knowledge. Many of Vennard's breathing exercises also fit well with current theory, although less emphasis is now placed on strength in the inhalation phase (Vennard uses heavy books on the belly, or encourages a solid thrust outwards of the epigastrium on inhalation) and more on flexibility and control of the out-breath through the abdominal musculature.

Vennard's text was considered a standard in vocal pedagogy for a number of years. His work is usually referred to in most singing texts since his time, although it is becoming less popular due, no doubt, to the publication of many other tomes. He can be seen as a significant influence on most of the American writers on vocal pedagogy since the 1960s.

Richard Miller is also considered one of the giants of singing pedagogy in the late twentieth and early twenty-first centuries. He has written numerous books on singing and teaching singing, perhaps the most well-known of which is his 1986 book, *The structure of singing: System and art in vocal technique*. Miller is a firm believer that breath management is vital to good singing. His books all provide insight into his beliefs about breathing and breath management in statements ranging from the simple, to the more detailed and complex such as:

'Breath management is the essential foundation for all skilled vocalism' (Miller, 2000, p. 32).

'In cultivated singing, thoracic, diaphragmatic, and abdominal aspects of respiration must be co-ordinated (dynamic muscle equilibrium) without exaggerated activity in any one of the three areas' (Miller, 1986, p. 23).

'Technical skill in singing is largely dependent on the singer's ability to achieve consistently that fine co-ordination of air flow and phonation – the vocal contest – which is determined by co-operation among the muscles of the larynx and the chest wall, and diaphragmatic contraction, a dynamic balancing between sub-glottic pressure and vocal fold resistance' (Miller, 1986, p. 23).

Miller is seen by many as a link between the older style of sensation- and imagery-based vocal pedagogy, and more up-to-date scientific knowledge. He believes that teachers must have accurate anatomical and physiological knowledge to teach well, and he claims to base his concepts about breathing on detailed anatomical and physiological fact, quoting frequently and heavily from classic anatomy sources such as *Gray's Anatomy* and from research in the 1960s by workers in acoustic phonetics, such as Ladefoged.

Miller, in all of his works, takes a uniform approach to breathing, support and breath management which he calls

'… appoggio (from the verb, appoggiare: to lean against, to be in contact with) is a form of breath management co-ordination that must be learned if the singer is to unite energy and freedom for successfully meeting the tasks of professional vocalism' (Miller, 2000, p. 32).

'Appoggio is a system for combining and balancing muscles and organs of the trunk and neck, controlling their relationships to the supraglottic resonators, so that no exaggerated function of any one of them affects the whole' (Miller, 1986, p. 23).

Miller states that appoggio is based on physical fact, related to the actions of the respiratory anatomy and physiology. He describes respiration in the following terms: on inspiration, the diaphragm contracts downwards and the expansion of the intercostals increases the volume of the lungs.

He believes that the action of the diaphragm is misunderstood by most singers, since the central tendon of the diaphragm is attached to the pericardium where the heart is housed. This means that the movement of the diaphragm is less than most singers think. Miller also states that the diaphragm is not locally controlled and that it is basically passive during expiration and phonation (Miller, 2000, p. 33). He suggests that in appoggio, the aim is to retain the inspiratory position of the sternum and ribcage for longer periods than in normal respiration, thus retarding the diaphragmatic ascent (Miller, 2000, p. 34).

Miller then begins to discuss the abdominal muscles and their involvement in the out-breath, stating that the singer's task is to develop dynamic rather than static equilibrium over the aerodynamic-myoelastic instrument (Miller, 2000, p. 38). His goal for efficient breath management is to allow the exiting air to be turned into tone through natural phonatory resistance. He believes that this process is stabilised via the appoggio, which does have its source in the antagonistic muscles of the abdominal wall. 'Appoggio relies on the natural antagonism of these muscles at the moment of inspiration.' (Miller, 2000, p. 39).

'For the tasks of singing it is necessary to retain the inspiratory gesture as long as possible and to reduce the increase of subglottic pressure that normally occurs during the expiratory gesture' (Miller, 2000, p. 40). He believes that the reduction of excessive air flow and the increase of subglottic pressure are achieved by remaining for as long as possible in the inspiratory gesture, so that the muscles of the torso are trained to delay the customary exhalation movement (Miller, 2000, p. 40).

In many ways, Miller is correct in his assessment of the situation. The airflow must be held constant and not be allowed to be too high when the lungs are full of air otherwise the singing tone would not be even, sustained and prolonged. His desire to stay in the position of inhalation is therefore sensible, but his method of achieving this has some problems. Requiring the abdominal/torso muscles to delay their natural exhalation movement will lead to excessive tension and a possible 'locking' of the abdominal wall. This could cause the respiratory system to be unbalanced and may lead to a reduction in airflow over the glottis, which could hamper rather than improve tone. Chapman (2006) believes that correct, physiologically accurate movement of the abdominal wall increases the intra-thoracic pressure, encouraging the diaphragm to maintain its action. The increase in the intra-thoracic pressure activates the mechano-pressure receptors in the intercostal muscles so that they continue their braking action for longer, reducing subglottic pressure and thus, sustaining and prolonging the tone.

It certainly appears that Miller, a pedagogue of high reputation, has an excellent vision for respiration during singing, but unfortunately some of his concepts for a breath management system are not consistent with current anatomical and physiological knowledge. Miller attempts to couch his breathing pedagogy in scientific terms, but more recent kinematic and EMG studies of singers do not support his premises. .

James McKinney is another member of the 'belly in' school of breathing. His book *The diagnosis and correction of vocal faults: A manual for teachers of singing and choir directors* was initially published in 1982 and then revised and somewhat expanded in 1994. McKinney also believes that breathing is a vital component of the singer's technique. In his introductory chapters he provides us with a number of systems to help classify vocal difficulties, one of which is 'according to the physical processes involved in the singing act: that is , (1) faults related to respiration, (2) faults related to phonation, (3) faults related to resonation and (4) faults related to articulation' (McKinney, 1994, p. 17). McKinney goes on to say that he has found this system of classifying faults based on physical processes the most convenient and logical. He also appears, by placing it as the first physical process to be examined, to be highlighting the importance of respiration in the act of singing. McKinney was himself a student of Vennard and the link between these two pedagogues is obvious. McKinney, because of his focus on faults in singing, has attempted to take the earlier work of Vennard further, but he is not always able to offer a better scientific basis for some of his statements.

McKinney provides a summary of normal respiration with basic anatomical and physiological information. He does not mention many of the respiratory muscles in detail but provides other sources that can be consulted. He states clearly that the diaphragm is the main muscle of inspiration and that expiration is a combination of elastic recoil forces and the action of the abdominal muscles. He describes respiration in correct anatomical and physiological terms, which he then links to his breathing pedagogy. He does make an interesting statement about the lungs, however, which supports the notion that abdomino-diaphragmatic breathing will be the most efficient for singing.

'The lower half of each lung is much better equipped with capillaries than the upper half. This means that the lower half is more efficient at taking oxygen out of the air and removing carbon dioxide from the blood stream'. (McKinney, 1994, p. 47).

McKinney also makes a clear distinction between natural or normal breathing, and breathing for singing. He believes that natural breathing has three stages: breathing in, breathing out, and rest or recovery, and that these stages are not under conscious control (McKinney, 1994, p. 48), whereas

'Breathing for singing has four stages (1) a breathing in period (inhalation), (2) a setting up controls period (suspension), (3) a controlled exhalation period (phonation), and (4) a recovery period; these stages must be under conscious control until they become conditioned reflexes. Many singers abandon conscious controls before their reflexes are fully conditioned and inherit chronic problems thereby'. (McKinney, 1994, p. 48).

McKinney believes that inhalation for singing is quicker than in natural breathing, and that a greater amount of air is inhaled. He also states that the inhaled breath goes deeper into the lungs (McKinney, 1994, p. 48). McKinney uses imagery to help the singer co-ordinate the conditioned reflexes that are needed for efficient breathing by providing what he calls, a 'proper mental preparation'. Images such as smelling a flower, pretending to begin to yawn, or pretending to drink a glass of water are used to help the singer breathe in correctly.

The use of imagery has long been used in singing pedagogy. The vocal instrument is impossible to see without special equipment, difficult to feel accurately, and has both voluntary (singing) and vegetative (eating and breathing) functions, which makes instruction by imagery almost a necessity. At the present time, we do not know if the images McKinney suggests actually make changes to the respiratory system's function, but it appears that they can be used to achieve a desired result. Interestingly, McKinney discusses the anatomy and physiology of each stage of the breath before presenting the images that he has found helpful in achieving these functions. This is quite different to singing pedagogues who provide the image and then attempt to justify it with anatomy.

McKinney also reminds us that postural considerations prior to breathing are important. 'The chest should be comfortably high, the lower abdomen comfortably in, and the upper abdomen free to move' (McKinney, 1994, p. 49).

McKinney's statements about the lower abdomen being comfortably in, prior to breathing, are somewhat unclear. It is most likely that he is requesting the singer to maintain core stability during the breathing cycle (the lower abdominal muscles being actively recruited for this task by being comfortably in). Or it could be that he is setting up the exhalatory phase by having tone in the lower abdominals in preparation for the co-ordinated effort of the entire abdominal region in the out-breath. He is certainly not advocating tightness or tension of the abdominal muscles, as evidenced by the following statement:

'When you inhale the breath seems to move into the body, down to the lungs and out around the middle of the body. This expansion around the middle of the body is both natural and desirable; it has been identified as the displacement of the abdominal organs by the descent of the diaphragm'. (McKinney, 1994, p. 49).

McKinney reaffirms physiological fact by reminding us that when the diaphragm moves down, there is expansion all around the body, but this expansion is greatest in the front of the body where there is greater elasticity. This frontal expansion is encouraged by the attachments of the diaphragm to the ribcage and spinal column, and the greater mobility of the abdomen at the front. McKinney also makes a point about pedagogues who believe that back, rib or lateral expansion is the main focus of the in-breath:

'Some teachers have made such a fetish of back expansion or rib expansion that the more normal frontal expansion is limited or even eliminated. This is a case of partial truth being established as the whole truth, which is an ever present danger in all facets of teaching singing'. (McKinney, 1994, p. 50).

The suspension phase of McKinney's breathing pedagogy has no correlate in natural breathing. Suspension occurs just prior to exhalation and McKinney believes that its purpose is to prepare the breath support mechanism for the phonation to follow (McKinney, 1994, p. 50). He also believes that this suspension allows 'an almost effortless inception of vocal tone without any major readjustment of the mechanism involved' (1994, p. 50). He goes on to state that since this suspension phase is not a part of natural breathing the singer must consciously acquire it.

Unfortunately, McKinney provides us with no scientific evidence for the suspension phase in the breath cycle for singing. Review of other literature also failed to find evidence for this component, although it may relate to the transitions between inspiration and expiration that were described by Watson and Hixon (1987), where there was a shift of volume from the abdomen to the ribcage just prior to phonation. Watson and Hixon describe this setting up of the system as being ready for phonation. However, it may also be that this portion of the respiratory cycle in singing has not been specifically evaluated. There is the possibility that the suspension phase becomes so rapid in fully trained singers, that it has escaped the attention of researchers who are not actively looking for it.

The controlled exhalation of the singer is vital for the maintenance of good tone. McKinney believes that the breath should be released quite slowly, as the diaphragm gradually releases its tension, so that the diaphragm acts as a releasing brake (McKinney, 1994, p. 50). He also states that the best way to achieve this gradual release of the diaphragm is to try to maintain the expansion around the middle of the body. This statement does seem at odds with current respiratory theory about exhalation, but McKinney then definitively states that the actual expansion around the middle of the body will decrease as the breath is expelled, with the abdominal girth significantly decreasing throughout the breath cycle. He maintains that the reduction in girth is so gradual that the singer always feels expanded (McKinney, 1994, p. 50). This is a good example of a pedagogical instruction based on sensation rather than fact.

McKinney is again attempting to use an image based on the feelings that many singers report, one of expansion, even though he acknowledges that the opposite actually does happen. This is consistent with the findings of Hixon and coworkers who discovered that singers' perceptions of how they breathed, and how they actually breathed during singing, were often at odds with each other (Hixon, 1987, p. 369). McKinney's suggestion that the diaphragm acts as a releasing brake is certainly diametrically opposed to Miller's belief, as Miller believes that the diaphragm relaxes as soon as inspiration is completed. Work as reported by Sundberg (1987), Leanderson and Sundberg (1988), and Watson et al. (1989) tends to support McKinney's view of the diaphragm as a releasing brake, particularly when the lung volumes are quite high.

McKinney's final phase of breathing for singing consists of recovery. McKinney desires a relaxation of all the muscles at the end of each breath so that tension is not increased or carried from one breath to another. It appears that there is a split second in time during which this relaxation occurs. Once the breath is expelled through the action of the abdominal muscles they release and, just prior to the activation of the diaphragm and its descent for the next in-breath, there would exist a state of relaxation. This relaxation phase would equate with the transition from expiration to inspiration noted by Watson and Hixon (1985). They believe that there is a reduction in the activity of the abdomen just prior to the reactivation of the diaphragm for the next in-breath. At that time, the ribcage is continuing its expiratory function, so there is a brief moment of paradoxical movement when the abdomen is assuming its inspiratory posture while the ribcage continues its expiratory work. The relaxation of the abdomen could be felt by the singer as an overall relaxation of the respiratory system prior to the next in-breath.

McKinney goes on to define breath support for singing as something slightly different from just inhalation and exhalation.

'Breath support is a dynamic relationship between the breathing in muscles and the breathing out muscles, the purpose of which is to supply adequate breath pressure to the vocal folds for the sustaining of any desired pitch or dynamic level. When a person establishes the correct posture, breathes in properly, and then suspends the breath, a balanced tension is set up between the muscles of inhalation and exhalation'. (McKinney, 1994, p. 53).

McKinney believes that, by trial and error, the singer learns to adjust this balanced tension as required. 'Only time and disciplined practice will bring the support mechanism to its full potential for supplying fine adjustments of breath pressure to the vocal folds' (McKinney, 1994, p 54).

McKinney makes an important point about breath support when he states that only time and disciplined practice will develop the support system fully. In the Bel Canto period, singers worked with a master for approximately seven years before being allowed to sing publicly. It can be postulated that, during this time, the breath support system was trained by a combination of instructions from the master, input from the sound produced, and by trial and error on the part of the singer.

McKinney completes his chapter on breathing and breath support by providing a summary of his breathing concepts. He states that the separate components of breathing must be brought together into a unified whole, and that breathing techniques need to be kept under conscious control until they become habitual.

Many singing pedagogues are attempting to change or modify their method of instruction about breathing based on the more current scientific research. Some teachers are now using almost purely mechanistic descriptions of the breath to help student singers towards an efficient breath management system for singing, while others use imagery and concepts to get physiological facts across to the student in a way that they can understand and use. Robert White (1988) believes that singing teachers have certain responsibilities in relation to scientific knowledge.

'Teachers of singing bear two major responsibilities. The first is to achieve a thorough understanding of the physiological-mechanical processes through which the singing voice is produced .... The second responsibility for teachers of singing is to formulate concepts [images] based on their understanding of the physiological-mechanical processes and present them to the students in terms they can understand and apply towards the development of a singing technique'. (White, 1988, p. 26).

White also reminds us that although there may be only one basic way for a breath to be taken or used, there are many ways of teaching these concepts, which can be driven by a changing imagery that is limited only by the teacher's imagination. White does not advocate teaching the action of every muscle to the student, but he does insist that the teacher has that knowledge to a level which allows him or her to produce meaningful, but physiologically correct images to help the student.

White's approach makes use of much of the current scientific research: he understands the connection between posture and breathing, he gives the diaphragm the role of prime mover for inspiration, with concomitant relaxation of the abdominal wall to allow its quick and easy descent, and also gives correct activity to the abdomen in its role of tuning the system and supporting the singing voice. White's model is easy to understand, and clearly follows the dictates of physiology. He goes on in his article to list the images he has found useful in achieving these aims. Similar to McKinney, he matches the images to the physiology, rather than attempting to match the physiology to the image.

There still seems to be difficulty in discarding some of the long held beliefs about breathing for singing even when scientific facts are clear. Leon Thurman states that:

> 'The profession of singing teaching is currently in a decades-long historic transition from pre-scientific vocal pedagogy to science-based voice education. During this transition, mixtures of pre-scientific and science-based concepts, terminologies, and practices are inevitable'. (Thurman, 2004, p. 28).

Thurman goes on to identify seven pre-scientific concepts about breathing that continue to exist and be used in voice studios today.

Concept One: 'There is a natural way to breathe for skilled speaking and singing, and it is involuntary' (Thurman, 2004, p. 30). This is the type of respiratory pattern that is used by infants. It is reasoned that if this natural type of breathing can be recovered or remembered, singing will be fine.

The main problem with this concept of breathing is the word 'natural'. Does natural mean prescribed by genetics? Does it mean physiologically most efficient? Certainly it is true that the respiratory system has a natural or physiologically driven way of behaving. Breathing strategies that are based on the body's own normal or natural functions are sure to be more efficient than those which are physiologically possible, but unusual or inefficient, or that use muscles whose prime functions are not respiratory.

While it is true that breathing for life (tidal breathing) is involuntary (we do it when asleep and it occurs even in the womb for practice), and that the rate and extent of breathing is regulated by the respiratory neurones based on the level of oxygen in the blood, not all breathing is involuntary. Breathing for vocalisation of any description requires a departure from this state. This becomes a breath which is voluntary. Thurman (2004) reminds us that although learned breathing co-ordinations can be experienced often enough to allow the details of their timing, sequence and intensity of muscle co-ordinations to be transferred to the subcortical motor areas of the brain, it is still the frontal cortex that initiates the required respiratory pattern at a chosen time, enabling the subcortical motor areas to enact the details (p. 34). This means, that once trained, the singer may feel that the breathing is essentially involuntary, as everything works correctly with merely the thought of the breath.

Singers need to develop breath management systems that follow the physiological rules of the respiratory system, and to practise those patterns until they become programmed into their subcortical motor systems, feeling almost involuntary.

Concept Two: 'Actions of the diaphragm muscle are involuntary and not subject to learned voluntary action' (Thurman, 2004, p. 30). Those who ascribe to this school of thought believe that the sensory innervation of the diaphragm does not allow the singer to obtain the necessary feedback for diaphragm control.

Although the diaphragm does not have sensory innervation that allows discrete control over the parts of the muscle, subtle variations in breath flow and pressure are required for singing. Thurman states that:

> 'One way that these subtle variations can be produced is to simultaneously co-contract (1) the abdominal muscles as one driving force for creation of lung-air pressure and breath flow, and (2) the thoracic diaphragm muscle as a checking force. This oppositional counterbalancing provides more potential for fine-tuned motor co-ordinations ....' (Thurman, 2004, p. 32).

This type of counterbalancing is in many ways an unnatural act and is learned, suggesting that proficient singers do have conscious control over the diaphragm, at least to some degree. This activity of the whole respiratory system with the inhalatory and exhalatory muscles working as a team is now well understood and certainly the well trained singer is able to use other parts of the respiratory system to help control the diaphragm.

Concept Three: 'During inhalation, the inhalation muscles of the lower ribs and back (e.g. external intercostals, latissimus dorsi) are prominently involved, while the abdominal and pelvic diaphragm muscles are passive' (Thurman, 2004, p. 30). The diaphragm's inhalatory action is admitted, but de-emphasised. This is the 'belly out' school of support, where exhalation is also supposed to be controlled with the muscles of the back, while the diaphragm and abdominal muscles are concerned with maintaining the 'belly out' posture. This viewpoint is really now quite unsustainable given our knowledge of the respiratory system both in quiet breathing and in breathing for speaking and singing.

Concept Four: 'A variant of the previous perspective [concept four] does emphasise diaphragm muscle action during inhalation with a passive expansion of the uncontracted abdominal muscles and a passive depression of the uncontracted pelvic diaphragm' (Thurman, 2004, p. 31). This variation of the 'belly out' school also insists that the abdominal and pelvic floor muscles do not control expiration; it is the role of the back and lower rib muscles, although the abdominal and pelvic diaphragm are thought to spring back passively during exhalation.

Both concepts three and four are relying on the use of the abdominal and pelvic floor muscles in their roles in defecation and expulsion of waste from the body, rather than in their roles as expiratory muscles. As McKinney points out, these styles of breathing tend to lock the diaphragm in its lower position. Thurman states that this prevents the diaphragm from performing its role as the main muscle of inhalation, particularly during inter-phrase breaths (Thurman, 2004, p. 34). There is also the issue that during forced defaecation and other types of exertion, the larynx is tightly closed to maintain the intra-thoracic pressure. This is not an efficient setting of the larynx for singing.

Concept Five: 'During inhalation, the ribcage is held 'up and open' in order to optimise (1) expansion of the lungs when the diaphragm muscle contracts to lower the thoracic diaphragm, and (2) outward movement of the lower ribs when their inhalation muscles are contracted' (Thurman, 2004, p. 31). During exhalation, the ribs are supposed to maintain their high posture, while the muscles of the abdomen contract the abdominal contents, pushing them up and expelling the air. As the air is expelled from the chest, lower rib muscles are also involved to maintain a steady flow. This is the 'belly in and up' school of support (Thurman, 2004, p. 31).

The use of concept five appropriately recruits the abdominal and pelvic floor muscles into their expiratory functions, but Thurman has some concerns that the demand for the high ribcage could distort the postural alignment of the singer, which is also not good for voice production. 'Typically, a 'hold the sternum up' instruction results in a contraction of spinal flexor muscles so that the upper chest and head are tilted backward and the lumbar and thoracic vertebrae of the spine become compressed together.' (Thurman, 2004, p. 35).

Concept Six: 'When singing, an optimum or balanced interactive co-ordination occurs between the postural and the respiratory muscles. This breathing co-ordination was described by Miller … and is conveyed in the Italian concept of appoggio [described above]' (Thurman, 2004, p. 31). Teachers in the appoggio school often inform students that when the breath is properly balanced, the abdomen and chest will not move very much and that there will be no sense of muscular work in the abdomen, merely a sense of 'tensile energy'.

Although the recommendation to have a sense of tensile energy in the abdomen and chest is a good one in that it can prevent the singer from using too much muscular force and over-pressurising the lungs, the insistence that the singer remain in the position of inhalation means that the ribcage, which is the major controller of breath pressure in singing, is prevented from participating in the generation of appropriate lung pressures (Thurman, 2004, p. 35). Miller, the most well known proponent of this method, states quite unequivocally that the diaphragm relaxes immediately after contraction and takes no real part in maintaining airflow, breath pressure or support. This does not agree with the concept that the diaphragm can perform the function of a releasing brake (checking force) against the action of the expiratory abdominal muscles.

This concept, that there is a balanced interaction between the postural muscles and the respiratory muscles, is an excellent one well grounded in physiological fact, but unfortunately, the details of this concept, how it is taught and how it is perceived do not continue to follow these physiological dictates.

Concept Seven: 'Good breath support and good breath connection are hallmarks of skilled singing' (Thurman, 2004, p. 31). Proponents of this concept often give only a broad instruction on breathing, such as 'you need to learn diaphragmatic breathing', 'breathe from your diaphragm', and 'breathe with your stomach muscles' (Thurman, 2004, p. 31).

Unfortunately, many of the techniques used by this school for the development of breathing are insufficiently specific. They may promote a better breath but because the actual process of breathing for singing is not properly explained, 'they all can lead to myth-conceptions about the process or they can lead to inefficiencies in other equally important voice co-ordinations' (Thurman, 2004, p. 35).

Many modern pedagogues are attempting, as White insists in his 1988 article, to use the newly acquired scientific knowledge to develop a breathing strategy that is not only physiologically accurate, fulfilling Thurman's criteria, but is also easy to teach and learn. Janice Chapman (2006) outlines a breathing and breath support system that is based not only on physiological fact but also has been trialled over a long period in her vocal studio.

Chapman believes that all singing should be supported by the muscles of the abdominal girdle and those that attach to the lower abdominal pubic symphysis (LAPS). She also believes that the diaphragm must be free and unhindered in its descent to allow full but natural inhalation for singing. In her pedagogy, inhalation is based on the 'SPLAT' manoeuvre. SPLAT has been described thus:

> 'Breathe out through pursed lips…as though through a drinking straw to the end of available breath without losing posture. Hold this position for a couple of seconds, while noticing where the tension is in the body - i.e. check with hands on waist band, xiphoid area (apex of sternum and ribs), and the lower abdominal/pubic symphysis (LAPS). Then release all tension and notice how the air is drawn in to the lungs automatically. The reason for this is that the diaphragm is free to contract and descend quickly, creating a vacuum in the lungs. Be aware of maintaining postural alignment during this release - i.e. if postural alignment is lost this rapid diaphragmatic descent is less efficient. This is the basis of the SPLAT breath'. (Chapman, 2006, p. 42)

In Chapman's pedagogy, the emphasis of control of the outward flow of air is with the abdominal and pelvic floor musculature. Immediately after the diaphragmatic in-breath, the singer is requested to draw the umbilicus in, thus activating the muscles of the abdominal girdle and LAPS and increasing the intra-abdominal pressure. The ribs are left free, not held in any specific position, so that they can control the pressurisation of the lungs. Chapman's pedagogy is consistent with many of the features of breathing for singing that were identified previously by Watson and Hixon (1987).

> 'In my pedagogy, the SPLAT in-breath is followed immediately by movement of the belly wall towards the spine, which brings about the activation of the abdominal girdle and LAPS. This raises the intra-abdominal pressure and the intra-thoracic pressure and is synchronised with the onset of phonation. This gives the singer the ability to use the compressed air with complete control. It is as though the singer has both accelerator (anterior abdominal wall and LAPS) and brakes (abdominal girdle, sides and back and, consequently, the diaphragm) under the same foot.' (Chapman, 2006, p. 41).

Chapman is also concerned about the interaction between the muscles of postural support and the muscles of respiration. She feels that there is significant interaction between these systems that can greatly influence the singer.

She then presents a set of exercises to promote the use of the respiratory physiology in the way that she has described. She uses the concept of primal sound to underpin her breathing technique. Primal sounds, such as laughing, crying, sobbing and wailing, are thought to be under the control of the emotional motor system. Production of these primal sounds calls on a response from the respiratory system that is neurologically hard-wired, based deep in our animal brain. The singer learns to develop control over these connections and muscular interactions by repeated stimulation of the link, raising the sensations to conscious awareness and practice of the required movements (Chapman, 2006).

In Chapman's pedagogy, respiratory muscles are called upon to act in accordance with their primary function. There is a scientific basis to the pedagogy. The interaction between breathing, support and posture is understood, and the breathing method does not interfere with other components of the vocal instrument.

Chapman also recommends some breathing exercises that can be carried out when not singing. Specifically, she suggests the use of the Accent Method to assist the student to make the necessary connections and to achieve the necessary practice to develop, strengthen, and co-ordinate the breath support system for singing.

Examining the approaches of a key group of pedagogues from the past five decades have shown that many changes have been made to the way in which they teach breathing, breath support or breath management. These changes in approach have been based on the research into breathing, and breathing for singing, carried out since the 1950s. However, some pedagogues continue to use pre-scientific images or concepts as the basis for their teaching. Others, for example Miller, use a type of pseudo-science, or are selective as to the attention they pay to scientific knowledge. It would appear that of the schools of breath management that were identified at the beginning of this chapter, only the 'belly in' school has a real scientific basis. The exact mechanism that should be used for singing is still uncertain, but any pedagogy that does not meet the criteria set out by Thurman (2004) can, on the basis of the findings in the previous chapter, be essentially discounted. The Accent Method, with its strong basis in science and its training aspect, can be considered a useful breath management strategy for singing. It falls within the 'belly in' school of singing and is actively encouraged by pedagogues such as Janice Chapman.

3

Accent Method principles and practice: speaking voice

The Accent Method is a training and treatment programme for the voice. It is well organised and extensively researched. A great strength of the Accent Method is its efficacy with both normal and disordered voices.

Core concepts in Accent Method

- Accent Method addresses the whole vocal system.

- It aims to optimise normal vocal function by training normal patterns of breathing and phonation.

- Accent Method works on achieving the co-ordination between breath voice and articulation.

- The exercises focus on abdomino-diaphragmatic breathing creating strength and flexibility in the abdominal muscles.

- The exercises should be in modal (M1) voice.

- The exercises build up in intensity and complexity. One stage is mastered before moving on to the next.

- Fricative sounds are used. They help to promote vocal fold closure with the least muscular tension in the vocal tract. They also allow monitoring of the airflow.

- The constant repetition promotes motor learning so that the breathing becomes automatic. Repetitive rhythms and breathing create a feeling of calm and assist with relaxation of the vocal tract.

- Research into the Accent Method suggests that it:

  - Normalises vocal fold closure

  - Normalises airflow

  - Increases dynamic range

  - Encourages flexibility and pliability of the vocal fold cover

  - Reduces oedema and mass-size changes of the vocal folds

  - Reduces muscle tension within the larynx and vocal tract

  - Reduces hard glottal attacks

'The Accent Method can be viewed as a technique to develop optimal voice and speech function by creating a perfect dynamic balance between subglottal air pressure and glottic activity, which will increase the acoustic flexibility of the voice' (Thyme-Frøkjær and Frøkjær-Jensen, 2001, p. 3). Although this is the stated aim for the speaking voice, it is even more applicable to the singing voice. Singers aim to have a delicate balance of subglottal air pressure and glottic activity to maintain pitch and loudness (Leanderson and Sundberg, 1988, p. 3), so any method that promotes this will be advantageous. Thyme-Frøkjær and Frøkjær-Jensen's other stated aims of the Accent Method are also appropriate to the requirements for singing. They claim that the Accent Method results in:

- A rich and beautiful timbre

- Excellent intelligibility with clear articulation

- Full dynamic range of soft to loud

- A lively intonation

- A voice that is sustainable through vocally stressful and challenging situations without succumbing to voice strain (Thyme-Frøkjær and Frøkjær-Jensen, 2001, p. 3).

The Accent Method claims to rely on sound physiological principles and has been described as a holistic and rational therapy.

> 'It is well known that efficient voice production is based upon the activity of the abdominal muscles. The Accent Method therefore uses exercises with a rhythmic change in the activity of these muscles as a central part in training. These exercises encourage control of the abdominal muscles to produce large or small contractions voluntarily'. (Thyme-Frøkjær and Frøkjær-Jensen, 2001, p. 3).

Given the results of experiments that have evaluated breathing for singing, it would appear that this type of voluntary control over the abdominal musculature would greatly assist the singer's breath management during singing.

The Accent Method was developed by Professor Svend Smith. Smith was a well-known speech pathologist and voice researcher in the 1920s and 1930s. It was from his extensive studies into speech physiology, and his knowledge of the theories and practices of the day, that in the 1930s, he saw a need for a new set of therapy activities for pathological voices (Thyme-Frøkjær and Frøkjær-Jensen, 2001, p. 5). Prior to 1935, most exercises for patients with voice disorders were based on the theories for singing training and on non-pathological voices, which Smith found ineffective for many of his patients. As a clinician, Smith had the luxury of trialling his new theory and practice on his patients, which quickly lead to an organised set of exercises.

> '...in 1937, his theory was formulated in detail and he was able to build up the complete system of treatment for pathological voices which incorporated: breathing exercises at rest, the transfer from expiration

at rest to expiration for phonation and various voice exercises matching the prosody of speech. A year later, an uncomplicated set of drum exercises was created which exactly fits the voice exercises'. (Thyme-Frøkjær and Frøkjær-Jensen, 2001, pp. 5–6).

Smith continued to consolidate his method through research and clinical practice and in 1967, the collaboration with Kirsten Thyme-Frøkjær began. Thyme-Frøkjær was particularly interested in the generalisation of the skills learnt by the patients in clinical voice training into spontaneous speech. She was instrumental in adding prosodic speech exercises that encouraged transfer of the skills through reading to spontaneous speech, and defined the main goal of the Accent Method as follows:

'to resolve pathological symptoms by optimising normal functions and to do this by achieving the best possible co-ordination between breathing, voicing, articulation, body movement and language for each individual'. (Thyme-Frøkjær and Frøkjær-Jensen, 2001, p. 7).

The Accent Method does not treat vocal pathology or inefficiency directly. Rather, it aims to train normal patterns of speech and voice production. It is this goal of training normal patterns of speech and voice production that makes the method so appropriate for singers. Studies into breathing for singing make it clear that the singers must use a natural, i.e., physiologically accurate and appropriate, breath for singing. The Accent Method, with its focus on training normal patterns including normal breathing patterns, is theoretically well suited for this purpose.

'The Accent Method relies on kinaesthetic feedback to control and co-ordinate body movement, breathing, phonatory and articulatory patterns' (Thyme-Frøkjær and Frøkjær-Jensen, 2001, p. 8). Initially, training begins with slow, gross movements that, once the client has sufficient control, are followed by quicker, finer movements. The Accent Method begins with minimal tension, which is considerably increased before returning to its original state. (Thyme-Frøkjær and Frøkjær-Jensen, 2001, p. 8).

> 'In normal, 'at rest' breathing, the body can be observed to move slightly forward during inhalation and slightly backwards during exhalation. These movements are produced automatically as the centre of gravity is shifted. During the breathing cycle, contraction of the diaphragm alternates with the contraction of the abdominal muscles. The pressure on the abdomen created by the contraction of the diaphragm moves the abdominal wall downwards and forwards during inhalation, thus shifting the centre of gravity forwards. During exhalation the abdominal muscles, in conjunction with the relaxation of the diaphragm, return the abdomen to its resting position, thus shifting the centre of gravity back again'. (Thyme-Frøkjær and Frøkjær-Jensen, 2001, p. 9).

Thyme-Frøkjær and Frøkjær-Jensen show the direct link between the Accent Method and the physiological facts, with an explanation that is consistent with the structure and function of the respiratory system as described by Hixon and others.

Accent Method exercises commence in a slow rhythm to train the correct abdominal breathing pattern, without any excessive muscular tension in the upper chest, and to allow sufficient time to develop a perfect balance between expiration, which creates the subglottal pressure, and the tension in the larynx which is required to resist that pressure for voicing (Thyme-Frøkjær and Frøkjær-Jensen, 2001, p. 9).

The fundamental principles of the Accent Method - that during the breathing cycle, contraction of the diaphragm alternates with contraction of the abdominal muscles and that training should move from slow, gross and more simple towards fast, fine and more complex - appear to be applicable to singing. Singing is a complex biomechanical process. Following the correct physiological dictates and building a technique from simple to complex should ensure a solid foundation for the expression of musical ideas.

The Accent Method has a defined set of exercises that move the student from breathing at rest to breathing for phonation.

Respiration at rest usually starts with the student in the supine position, with a small pillow or books under the neck if required to enhance comfort. At this stage, very little instruction is given to the student. Merely placing the body in the correct posturally aligned position will usually result in natural abdomino-diaphragmatic breathing. The student may be told that breathing can be seen as a three part action, with inspiration, expiration and a pause. In reality, there is no pause between inspiration and expiration, but as expiration usually takes twice as long as inspiration, the student will easily accept as a pause the decrease in effort as the expiration transitions into the next inspiration (Thyme-Frøkjær and Frøkjær-Jensen, 2001, p. 95). Once abdomino-diaphragmatic breathing is established, the student is made consciously aware of it by placing one hand on the abdomen to feel the rise and fall of the abdomen, which occurs in each breath cycle.

The student can also be made aware of the lack of movement in the upper chest during a correct abdomino-diaphragmatic breath by placing the other hand on the upper chest and noting the lack of movement there in contrast to the active movement in the abdomen (Thyme-Frøkjær and Frøkjær-Jensen, 2001, p. 95).

The student is then requested to make a breathy /w/ sound on the outgoing airstream; this is a transitional stage between breathing at rest and breathing for speech. At this stage, in the supine position, inspiration is active, under the control of the diaphragm, while expiration is passive and predominantly driven by the elastic recoil of the respiratory system (Thyme-Frøkjær and Frøkjær-Jensen, 2001, p. 96).

'When the exercises in the supine position are mastered, the same exercise can be carried out while lying on the side, which is somewhat more difficult than in the supine position, because in this position the weight of the abdominal content does not support the expiration and therefore the abdominal muscles must be somewhat active'. (Thyme-Frøkjær and Frøkjær-Jensen, 2001, p. 96).

Once the exercises can be performed to a satisfactory level of efficiency in the side lying position, the student is moved onto a stool or a straight-backed chair. More active involvement of the abdominal muscles will be required for all the expiratory exercises, as gravity no longer assists expiration but assists inspiration instead. The next stage is in the standing position, with the addition of some body movements (Thyme-Frøkjær and Frøkjær-Jensen, 2001, p. 98).

In the standing position, to facilitate the exercise and to emphasise natural breathing, the student is encouraged to allow the body to move slightly backwards and forwards as the centre of gravity shifts. The student is also encouraged to breathe deeply, without lifting or over tensing the chest (Thyme-Frøkjær and Frøkjær-Jensen, 2001, p. 99).

Voiced exercises are introduced once respiration is firmly established in the standing position, at rest. The phonation that is used is low and breathy to promote improved elasticity and flexibility of the mucosa. Each exercise is performed with low intensity in the beginning, increased intensity in the middle and, again, with low intensity at the end (Thyme-Frøkjær and Frøkjær-Jensen, 2001, p. 106). Dr Nasser Kotby suggests that voiceless and voiced fricatives can be used here, almost as a pre-phonatory stage, to ensure that the airflow is sufficiently high. He also suggests using these fricatives to develop appropriate accentuations (Kotby, 1995, p. 63). Once this is established, the first set of the true rhythmic exercises can be commenced. These are usually trained on close vowels with a slightly breathy voice quality to ensure that there is no excessive tension in the articulators or larynx. Largo exercises are usually performed at about 58 beats per minute (Thyme-Frøkjær and Frøkjær-Jensen, 2001, p. 108).

Tempo I, Variation I

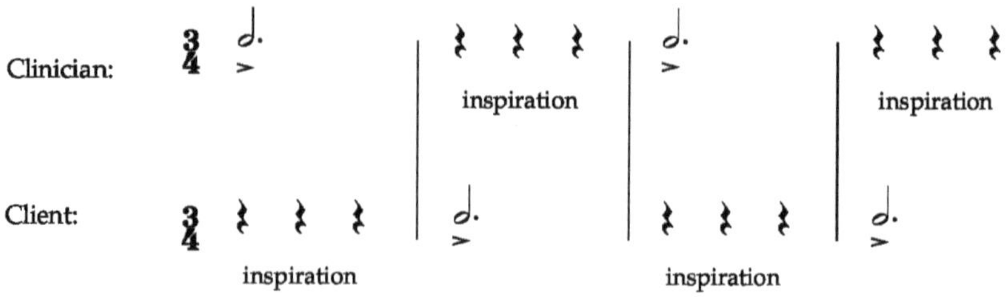

Tempo I, Variation 2

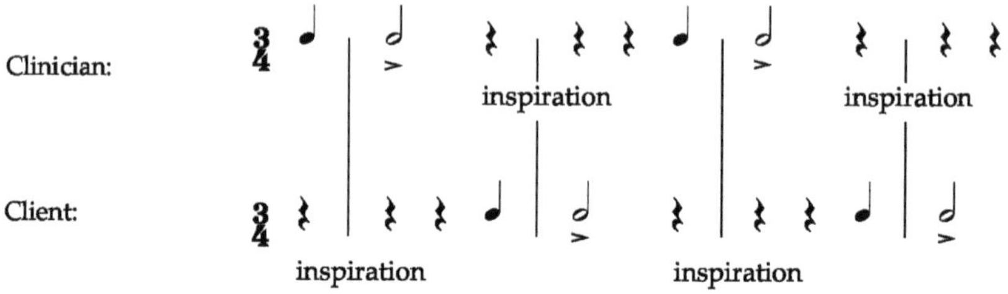

Tempo I, Variation 3

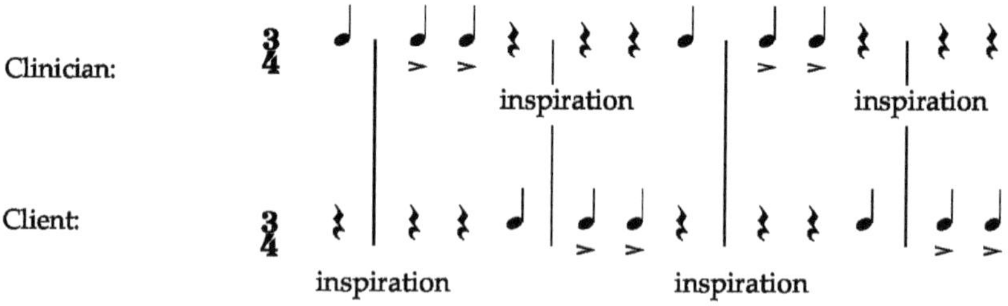

Figure 3.1 Rhythmic notation for the three patterns of Largo (Tempo I) as described in Thyme-Frøkjær, K. & Frøkjær-Jenson, B., 2001, p. 106 and p. 110.

As the other patterns in Largo (the first tempo) are introduced, the 'voice quality will be changed to a clear and sonorous timbre, with distinct articulation and without any signs of breathiness or glottal fry' (Thyme-Frøkjær and Frøkjær-Jensen, 2001, p. 109). As the airflow is controlled voluntarily by the student, a change in the movement of the whole chest wall can be discerned.

> 'In contradistinction to the respiration at rest, where the chest must not move, it is important that the chest moves upwards during the accentuated phonation. But this movement must always be a passive one, caused exclusively by the compression of the air in the lungs during the abdominal muscle contraction necessary for the accentuated phonation. This movement can be observed in the exercises as a raising of the sternum during each accentuation' (Thyme-Frøkjær and Frøkjær-Jensen, 2001, p. 109).

Arm and body movements can also be added to the Largo patterns to assist the airflow out of the lungs and to activate the accentuated voice patterns. The quiet inspiration and calm swinging rhythm with the arms is also thought to promote relaxation (Thyme-Frøkjær and Frøkjær-Jensen, 2001, p. 111).

Once the student has good control over the respiratory function and has an improvement in the sonority of the vocal timbre, the second rhythmic pattern of Andante can be introduced.

Andante is essentially a march rhythm with four beats to the bar. The exercise usually begins at around 70 beats per minute but may be gradually increased to 80 beats per minute (Thyme-Frøkjær and Frøkjær-Jensen, 2001, p. 113). The exercises are performed with a quick inspiration followed by an unaccentuated upbeat which precedes the accentuated beats. 'Variations in Tempo II [Andante] are introduced to reinforce co-ordination between respiration, phonation and articulation, and to promote general elasticity and mobility' (Thyme-Frøkjær and Frøkjær-Jensen, 2001, p. 113).

Tempo II, Variation I

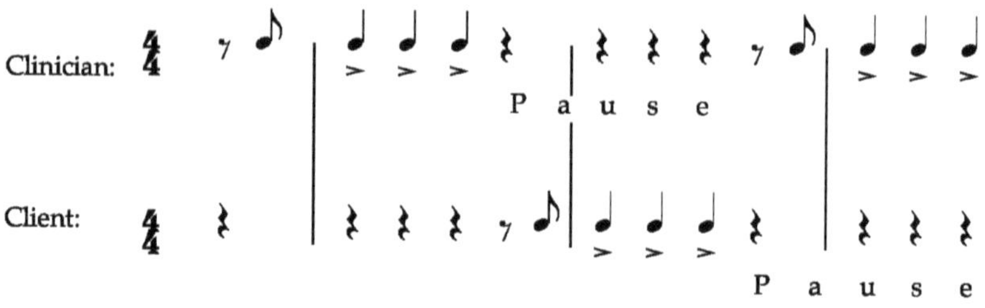

Tempo II, Variation 2

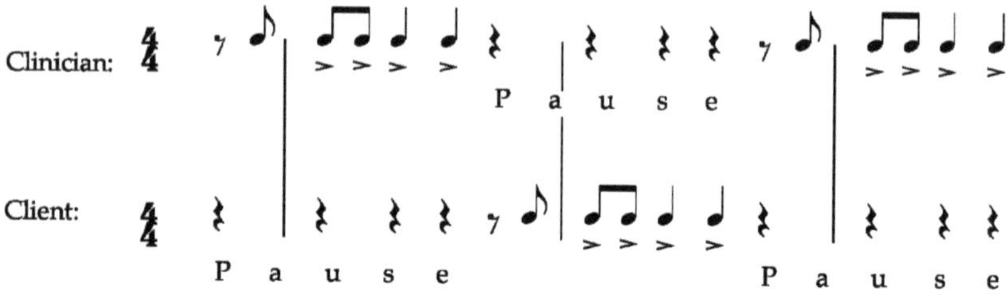

Tempo II, Variation 3

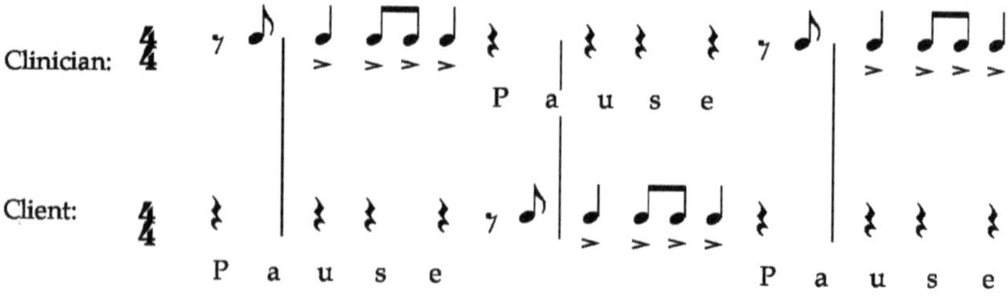

Figure 3.2 Rhythmic notation for the three patterns of Andante (Tempo II) as described in Thyme-Frøkjær, K. & Frøkjær-Jenson, B. 2001, p. 114 and p. 115.

Once again, arm and body movements can be added to the exercises to assist accentuation and develop strength and flexibility.

Tempo III, or Allegro, has four beats to the bar, as does Andante, but the tempo is somewhat faster at about 88 beats per minute. The main difference between Andante and Allegro is that the first two beats of each bar are subdivided. The entire exercise consists of a short and deep active inspiration directly followed by an unaccentuated eighth [quaver] as an upbeat, four accentuated eighths and an accentuated quarter [crotchet]' (Thyme-Frøkjær and Frøkjær-Jensen, 2001, p. 116).

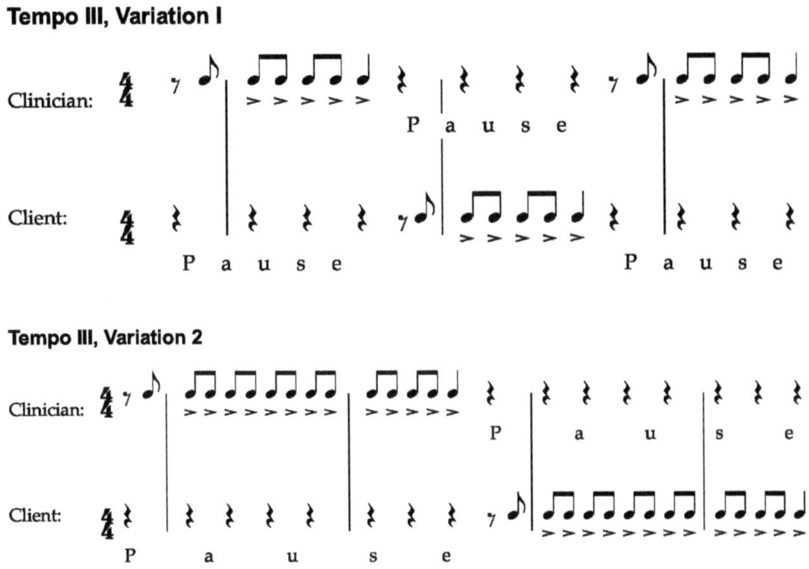

Tempo III, Variation 1

Tempo III, Variation 2

Figure 3.3 Rhythmic notation for the three patterns of Allegro (Tempo III) as described in Thyme-Frøkjær, K. & Frøkjær-Jenson, B. 2001, p. 116 and p. 117

Thyme-Frøkjær and Frøkjær-Jensen point out that the purpose of the Allegro patterns is to increase the number of accentuations on each breath. 'By training rapid strings of accentuations the client or actor also trains the mobility and fine co-ordination of respiration, phonation and articulation' (2001, p. 117).

'In tempo III variations, the single movements of the abdominal wall and the chest cannot be seen clearly, because the number of accentuations follow quickly after each other. Therefore the two variations described will be seen rather as a continuous inward movement of the abdominal wall and a continuous, weaker outward movement of the chest' (Thyme-Frøkjær and Frøkjær-Jensen, 2001, p. 118).

Body and hand movements can again be added to the Allegro patterns, but it is also possible to combine the patterns of both Andante and Allegro patterns since both are based on a 4/4 march time. Classically, the Accent Method has concentrated on using closed vowels initially, followed by the more open vowels, and then consonant-vowel babble. Thyme-Frøkjær and Frøkjær-Jensen also indicate that some of the voiced fricatives such as /z/ or /v/, or other voiced consonants such as /j/, can also be used in place of the closed vowels (2001, p. 11).

Once the voice and respiratory movements are correct in all of the tempos, work can be commenced, with words and phrases as a bridge into reading aloud texts and transfer into spontaneous speech. Thyme-Frøkjær and Frøkjær-Jensen state that the enhancement of prosody also improves articulation and intelligibility. The rhythmic patterns should be modified to fit the patterns of speech, but a connection to the accentuated vowels and consonant-vowel babble is maintained (2001, p. 128).

The course of instruction in the Accent Method is clearly defined and the hierarchy of tasks is also well ordered. These are some of the major deficits with other types of breathing instruction. In revisiting the results of scientific work on singing, and the requirements for a breathing pedagogy that arose from them, it can be seen that the Accent Method, because of its focus on abdomino-diaphragmatic breathing, voluntary control of respiration and repetitive rhythmic exercises, is able to fulfil these requirements well. The use of the repetitive exercises, first with closed vowels or fricatives and later with vowels and consonant-vowel babble, ensures high breath flow and gradual strengthening of the respiratory muscles. The use of rhythm also encourages the development of coordination and flexibility.

The Accent Method gives singers the necessary repetitive practice to allow the development of the fine interactions between inhalation and exhalation that constitute breath support. Singers are also given specific instructions to encourage development and use of the necessary muscles in the abdomen. This allows the abdomen to take its function in tuning the respiratory system for action, while allowing the rib cage to be free to control the pressurisation of air within the respiratory system. It could also be postulated that the exercises could aid the development of the function of the diaphragm as a releasing brake.

Kotby stresses that the training of breathing is considered to be the basis of the Accent Method. He also points out that the Accent Method actively trains respiratory support by focusing on the abdominal control of the outgoing airstream. 'Co-activation of the abdominal and flank muscles is, however, the main target of the expiratory exercises used in the Accent Method. These exercises are effective in reaching the goals of better respiratory support'. (Kotby, 1995, p. 57).

Research into the Accent Method

The Accent Method has been extensively studied both in clinical populations of patients with disordered voices and in those who have undergone training programmes for the teaching of the Accent Method. Thyme-Frøkjær and Frøkjær-Jensen have recorded some 400 clinicians, students of logopaedics (speech therapy), and large numbers of dysphonic patients. The recordings and analyses of the normal voices were made in connection with intensive courses, workshops and regular training in the Accent Method and therapy (Thyme-Frøkjær and Frøkjær-Jensen, 2001, p. 144). The recordings and studies performed on subjects who had normal larynges provides some insight into the possible changes that could occur in the voices and breath management systems of young singers. In all likelihood, the subjects for this present study will have normal larynges.

Thyme-Frøkjær and Frøkjær-Jensen reported on two studies of vital capacity and peak flow measures made before and after a one week intensive Accent Method course. They found a significant increase in the peak flow rate (measured in litres per second) for both studies following the Accent Method course. This would suggest that the subjects were better able to make sudden and strong contractions of the abdominal and chest muscles following this short but intensive training programme (2001, p. 145). Although vital capacity measures only improved significantly in one of the two study groups, there was a clear tendency towards improvement. Thyme-Frøkjær and Frøkjær-Jensen concluded:

'Thus improved respiratory function is shown by a minor increase in the vital capacity and by an increased peak airflow rate; that is, both the lung capacity and the ability to make a sudden strong expiratory muscle contraction are increased during the therapy'. (Thyme-Frøkjær and Frøkjær-Jensen, 2001, p. 146).

In another series of studies, recordings were made using electro-glottography in a class of 15 students who were studying speech therapy. They received Accent Method training over a 10 month period and duty cycle measures were obtained from the electroglottographic recordings. The duty cycle measure provides an estimation of the closed phase of the vocal folds' vibration cycle. Prior to training, the students' voices were evaluated subjectively as either hypofunctional (breathy) in 10 students or hyperfunctional (pressed or creaky) in five. All the students had normal healthy larynges according to their otolaryngologist. Following Accent Method training, the duty cycle for the hypofunctional voices had decreased (suggesting improved vocal fold closure) while those of the hyperfunctional students had increased (suggesting looser closure). Unfortunately, due to limited numbers in the hyperfunctional group, these data were not statistically significant. Thyme-Frøkjær and Frøkjær-Jensen concluded that:

'The balance between subglottal air pressure and vocal fold activity is adjusted to the greatest efficiency in relation to the energy used; that is, hypofunctional voices get a longer closure phase and hyperfunctional voices get a shorter closure phase'. (Thyme-Frøkjær and Frøkjær-Jensen, 2001, p. 147).

Thyme-Frøkjær and Frøkjær-Jensen also reported on data from a group of female clinicians who were rated as having hypofunctional voices prior to an intensive Accent Method course. They showed similar reductions in the duty cycle of the electroglottogram, but they also showed a significant reduction in mean airflow rate through steady state vowels. This was accompanied by a small but statistically significant increase in maximum phonation time. Mean flow rate dropped from 173 ml/s to 137 ml/s, where mean flow rates between 100 and 140 ml/s are considered normal (Thyme-Frøkjær and Frøkjær-Jensen, 2001, p. 149). Maximum phonation times increased from 20 s to 21.5 s. These changes occurred over the duration of a one week intensive Accent Method course.

> 'The main effect of the training of the phonatory system is improved balance between the expiratory activity (the airflow and subglottal air pressure) and the adjustment of the vocal folds (tension, thickness, length and adduction). This is due partly to improved mobility and elasticity of the vocal fold tissue and mucous membranes, and a better fixation of the mucous membrane to the underlying tissue, and partly to improved control of the respiratory and phonatory muscles taking part in voice production caused by the unconscious training of the feedback loops used for speech production'. (Thyme-Frøkjær and Frøkjær-Jensen, 2001, p. 150).

Thyme-Frøkjær and Frøkjær-Jensen report significant acoustic changes in voices post Accent Method training. They studied 20 clinicians who attended an initial week of an intensive Accent Method course and who then returned 12–24 months later to take part in an advanced course. They found significant changes in their phonetograms (a measure of the softest and loudest volume at each semitone of the pitch range) following the initial training course, with an average increase in total pitch range of 3.3 semitones and an increase in the dynamic range of 10.6 dB (Thyme-Frøkjær and Frøkjær-Jensen, 2001, p. 150). When the phonetograms were taken again 12–24 months after the initial course, it was found that again, there was some increase in both pitch and dynamic range. It appears that the effects of the Accent Method are maintained well over a lengthy period, though it must be noted that these clinicians did continue to train and treat patients in their own clinical practice, meaning that they were regularly practising the Accent Method in the gap between recordings.

The results of these studies, performed on subjects with essentially normal speech and voice production suggest that the Accent Method is able to enhance both respiratory and phonatory function, even if no significant vocal pathology is evident. This provides solid evidence for the claim that the Accent Method trains normal functions of respiration, phonation and articulation by enhancing the strength, efficiency and co-ordination of movement in the respiratory and phonatory systems.

The efficacy of the Accent Method has also been studied in relation to pathological or disordered voices. Kotby reported on his study (Kotby *et al.*, 1991) which examined a number of aerodynamic and perceptual measures that were taken before and after Accent Method therapy. They studied patients with non-organic (functional) voice disorders, vocal nodules and vocal cord paralyses. Following 20 sessions of the Accent Method, they found significant positive changes to voice quality in most of their patients. This perceptual improvement was also mirrored in the aerodynamic measures, with significant improvement in maximum phonation time, mean flow rate, subglottal pressures and glottal efficiency. 'Kotby *et al.* (1991) concluded that the Accent Method is therapeutically effective in non-organic (functional) voice disorders, vocal nodules and paralysis of the vocal folds' (Kotby, 1995, p. 85).

Fex *et al.* (1994) evaluated the efficacy of the Accent Method in patients with functional voice disorders. They examined a series of 10 consecutive patients who were referred to the speech pathologist. Seven patients had normal larynges, while three had moderate sized vocal nodules. They assessed a number of acoustic parameters: pitch perturbation quotient, amplitude perturbation quotient, normalised noise energy for 0–4 kHz and for 1–4 kHz, fundamental frequency and level differences. Patients were given 10, 30-minute Accent Method sessions, the timing of which necessarily varied according to patient requirements. Statistically significant changes were noted in pitch perturbation quotient and amplitude perturbation quotient for all the subjects. Normalised energy changes in the 1-4 kHz range and in fundamental frequency were statistically significant for the female patients only. These results confirm that the Accent Method is effective in making changes to pathological voices. The changes in the acoustic parameters towards more normal values agreed with the perceptual analysis of the voices that also suggested improvements. The Accent Method, by increasing airflow and normalising vocal fold function, was able to make statistically significant changes to a number of acoustic measures.

Bassiouny (1998) also studied the efficacy of the Accent Method. He used 42 patients who presented with a variety of vocal pathologies. Patients were randomly assigned to one of two treatment groups. Group one received Accent Method instruction in addition to advice about vocal hygiene, while group two received vocal hygiene advice only (they were scheduled to receive active voice treatment at a later date). Apart from the auditory perceptual analysis and videostroboscopic examination, all the patients were assessed with a number of acoustic and aerodynamic measures. Patients were assessed pre-therapy, half way through therapy, and post-therapy.

Aerodynamic measures consisted of: vital capacity, maximum phonation time, phonatory quotient, mean flow rate, subglottal pressure, glottal efficiency and a phonetogram. Acoustic analysis included: average pitch, pitch and amplitude perturbation quotients and the harmonic to noise ratio.

Auditory perceptual analysis results suggested that patients in the treatment group showed a greater degree of improvement that those in the hygiene only group. Similarly, videostroboscopic findings were highly significant in favour of the treatment group, with the hygiene-only group showing no significant changes in stroboscopy data (Bassiouny, 1998, p. 153).

'The difference in improvement of aerodynamic measures between pre- and post-test evaluation of both groups was highly significant in favour of the first group in the following parameters: SPL range [phonetogram data], subglottal pressure, glottal efficiency and glottal resistance' (Bassiouny, 1998, p. 154). Other aerodynamic measures showed significant improvements depending on the aetiology of the vocal disorder; hyperfunctional voices showed significant improvements in mean airflow, while the vocal fold paralysis group showed increased maximum phonation time, mean flow rates and a greater phonation quotient consistent with better vocal fold approximation. 'There was a non-conformity of improvement in all three parameters of acoustic analysis between the groups. The aetiological subgroups showed an additional inconsistency in the trend of improvement among the computed parameters of acoustic analysis' (Bassiouny, 1998, p. 163). Bassiouny believes that the lack of consistency in the acoustic data may be because the measures taken were not sensitive or specific enough (1998, p, 163). Overall, Bassiouny concluded that the treatment group who had the Accent Method exercises in addition to the vocal hygiene advice showed significantly greater improvement.

The results of studies on the efficacy of the Accent Method, both with normal and pathological voices, suggest that it is an effective tool for voice change. A significant improvement in the volume and pitch ranges (phonetograms) and a normalisation of parameters, such as mean airflow, vocal fold closure, glottal efficiency and subglottic pressure, have been reported. Pathological voices also often show changes in acoustic parameters, such as frequency and amplitude perturbation quotients and fundamental frequency, depending on the aetiology of the voice disorder.

The positive results obtained with subjects who had normal voices or larynges are of particular interest to teachers, singers and students of singing. Singers need to produce their voices in as efficient way as possible, over a wide variation of pitches and volumes. It appears that Accent Method exercises can assist them in the acquisition of these skills.

Unfortunately, no studies had been published that evaluated the use of the Accent Method for developing good respiratory (breath management and breath support) habits for singing, but it would appear, when evidence from studies into breathing for singing are taken into account, that the Accent Method would be a valuable pedagogical tool. In her 2006 book, Janice Chapman certainly uses Accent Method exercises, albeit slightly modified, as the basis of her breathing and support technique.

4

Modifications to the Accent Method for singing

Much of the classic Accent Method works well for singing. The most important aspects of method carry over into singing with few modifications.

Advantages of the Accent Method breathing for singing:

- It works on the whole vocal system
- It develops abdomino-diaphragmatic breathing
- It promotes good vocal fold closure
- It develops strength, flexibility and endurance
- It balances muscle and breath energy
- It helps give fine control over the abdominal muscles
- It promotes co-ordination of breath and voice
- It increases the dynamic range of the voice
- The repetitive nature of the exercises encourages unconscious learning
- The breathing patterns become automatic
- It promotes freedom and relaxation throughout the whole vocal tract.

However, some adjustments are needed for singing. The main difference is that singing requires extra muscular energy, commonly known as support. Classic Accent Method trains the muscles gently over time, but for singing it is necessary to introduce more muscular energy directly.

Sounds such as laughing, crying, groaning or calling help the singer feel the muscle activity that will be required later. This muscle connection will need to be added and is thus an integral part of the exercises for a singer.

In the classic Accent Method, close vowels are often used. For singers, we tend to use the fricatives more. This is because:

- They are semi-occluded vocal tract sounds. They create back pressure, encouraging good vocal fold closure

- They have a higher airflow than vowel sounds

- They make it easier to monitor the airflow

- They help connect to the support system while keeping the throat open.

In the Accent Method, the in-breath is initially extended to the same length as the out-breath. We have found that this can be counter-productive when working with singers, particularly if they over-breathe and become tense. We prefer to use a short inhalation from early on in the training. The in-breath is merely the recoil or response to having breathed out. It is important for the singer to be able to breathe in quickly and efficiently. The support muscles should not be engaged during the in-breath. The in-breath itself is not the performance!

In singing, we are required to manage the breath over much longer phases than in speaking. Using more complex rhythms helps extend the breath and gain finer control. The principles of moving from slow to faster, and simple to more complex, remain vitally important and the early stages should not be rushed through. Once the initial stages are mastered, singers will benefit most by working through more complex rhythms.

IF IN DOUBT, BREATHE OUT!

It is often said that men and women breathe differently. In fact, the respiratory anatomy and physiology are the same for both men and women. There are, however, differences in the structure and function of the pelvic floor. When doing abdomino-diaphragmatic breathing, men will feel the movement of the abdominal wall more around the navel, whereas women will feel it lower down. When teaching the Accent Method to singers, it is important to bear this in mind. When monitoring breathing, we suggest placing the thumb on the navel with the fingers on the lower abdomen. This will ensure adequate feedback, regardless of gender!

5

Research into the Accent Method for the singing voice

This research was undertaken as part of a Ph.D. study. Although some singers and singing teachers have used the Accent Method as part of their breathing pedagogy, there has been no specific research into the efficacy of the method with the singing voice.

The Accent Method had been taught as part of the principal practical study of classical voice at the Queensland Conservatorium of Music at Griffith University (QCGU), Australia, for a number of years. Both the vocal professors and the students felt that the course of the Accent Method was beneficial. These anecdotal reports of benefit prompted the design and implementation of the study.

If you want more detailed information regarding the research, including the statistics and graphs, please read on!

As a guide, when statistical analyses are made, scores are considered significant when:

- $p = 0.05$ level, there is a 95% chance that the result is 'real'

- $p = 0.01$ level is considered highly significant. There is a 99% chance that the score is 'real'.

In an experimental study of this type, a significant or highly significant score would suggest that any differences would be due to the training (i.e. Accent Method).

Core concepts in Accent Method research

The study was a two group design:

- An experimental group received Accent Method instruction
- A control group received no Accent Method instruction

Following 10 weeks of Accent Method instruction in a group class, there were some significant differences between measurements in the experimental group.

- A very significant increase in the dynamic range, that is, the difference between the softest and loudest tones sung, was seen for the experimental group. This was not so in the control group.

- After training the experimental group had a significantly wider pitch range than before training.

- Abnormal air flow traces became more normal after Accent Method instruction.

- Four subjects in the experimental group had abnormal airflow tracings before training. Only one showed this after training.

The control group had five subjects with abnormal tracings at the beginning of the study. At the end of the study, there were two additional subjects with abnormal tracings, making a total of seven. These students had been, or were being, taught either 'belly out' or 'belly neither one nor the other' for breath management.

Trained judges (singing professors at a tertiary institution) preferred the singing of the experimental group after training than before. They did not show this preference for the control group.

There was no change in the maximum phonation time, or mean airflow in either group post -training.

Overall, the Accent Method was felt to be effective in improving the voices of young classical singing students.

The study was carried out to quantify the anecdotal reports of improvements and the efficacy of a 10-week Accent Method course. The study used 30 classical singing students in their first or second year from the Guildhall School of Music and Drama in London, where, at that time, the Accent Method was not routinely taught. The study was a simple two group design in which the experimental group received Accent Method instruction and the control group was seen for the same amount of time, but was given sight reading rather than Accent Method instruction. The two groups underwent a series of measurements before and after training to evaluate any differences that occurred. Both groups of students continued their usual timetable, including individual voice lessons throughout the period.

Based on the findings of Thyme-Frøkjær on normal speaking voices, four main measurements were taken:

- Maximum Phonation Time (MPT) on the vowels /a/and /i/ at modal speaking pitch

- Aerodynamic studies (consisting of mean flow rates through steady state vowels /a/ and /i/ at modal pitch and one octave above modal pitch)

- A phonetogram (the students sang every semitone in their vocal range as softly and then as loudly as possible)

- A perceptual judgement (where singing teachers rated a section of 'Caro Mio Ben' by Giordani) sung unaccompanied in the key chosen by the student's vocal professor.

The subjects were randomly assigned to either the control or the experimental group. The groups were balanced for males and females and for first and second year students. Following the participant selection process, 29 participants were included in the study, 14 in the control group and 15 in the experimental group.

At the initial assessment, all of the subjects undertook a standard perceptual voice rating protocol to ensure that at the beginning of the study they had normal voices. No subject had abnormal scores and all were able to participate. Table 5.1 shows the demographic breakdown of the experiment.

Table 5.1 Demographics

Group/Demographic	Control	Experimental
Age Range	18 – 23	18 – 25
Males	6	7
Females	8	8
First Year	6	9
Second Year	8	6

The demographic characteristics of the two groups are essentially balanced (Table 5.1), although there are three more first year singers in the Experimental group ($N = 29$. Control: $n = 14$. Experimental: $n = 15$).

A t-test for equality of means (Table 5.2) was then performed to identify any significant differences between the two groups in terms of vocal function characteristics. There was only one significant difference identified. The MPT of the /i/ vowel was longer in the control group than in the experimental group at the $p < 0.05$ level of significance. All other pairs of results evaluated showed no significant differences and the groups were felt to be appropriately randomised and equivalent prior to the experiment.

Table 5.2 Assessment levels for different measures for the Control and Experimental group at initiation with differences assessed using Independent t-tests

Measurement	Group	M	SD	t	df	Sig. (2-tailed)
MPT /a/	Control	20.33	6.01	1.240	27	0.226
	Experimental	17.94	4.30			
MPT /i/	Control	23.34	6.86	2.081*	27	0.47
	Experimental	18.93	4.37			
Av DR	Control	21.56	5.90	−0.020	27	0.984
	Experimental	21.61	6.32			
Max Semi	Control	37.57	3.48	1.631	27	0.115
	Experimental	35.73	2.55			
MFR /a/	Control	155	69	−0.170	26	0.866
	Experimental	159	55			
MFR /a/8va	Control	243	77	−0.585	26	0.564
	Experimental	265	117			
MFR /i/	Control	153	74	−0.732	26	0.471
	Experimental	171	54			
MFR /i/8va	Control	223	72	0.088	26	0.931
	Experimental	220	104			

Note: MPT = maximum phonation time in seconds.
Av DR = average dynamic range in decibels.
Max Semi = maximum number of semitones sung.
MFR = mean flow rate in ml/s.
8va = one octave above modal pitch. * = $p < 0.05$.

Significant findings

Aerodynamic studies

The normative values for mean flow rates (MFR), taken in a steady state vowel /a/ at modal pitch, have been reported by Thyme- Frøkjær (2001) as 120 ml/s ± 20, giving a normal range of 100 to 140 ml/s. Initial assessment of the subjects in this study suggested a significantly higher value, as can be seen below.

Table 5.3 Mean flow rate in millilitres per second for all the subjects pre- and post-training

Condition	M	SD	t	df	Sig (2-tailed)
/a/ Modal Pre	152	57	−5.069***	26	0.000
/a/ 8va Pre	254	101			
/i/ Modal Pre	159	61	−3.515 **	26	0.002
/i/ 8va Pre	222	90			
/a/ Modal Post	168	50	−6.845 ***	27	0.000
/a/ 8va Post	248	74			
/i/ Modal Post	176	63	−3.271 **	27	0.003
/i/ 8va Post	224	83			

Note. ** = $p < 0.01$, *** = $p < 0.001$.

MFRs were significantly higher in the whole group than those reported by Thyme-Frøkjær (2001). The averages reported for the whole group are higher at both the pre- and post-training assessments.

MFRs were significantly higher for the vowels sung one octave above modal pitch. This difference occurred at both assessment points. However, there were no significant differences between the /a/ and /i/ vowels.

Table 5.4 Mean flow rates in millilitres per second in experimental and control groups pre- and post-training

Group/Task	*M*	*SD*	*t*	*df*	Sig (2-tailed)
Control					
/a/ Modal Pre /a/ Modal Post	155 183	70 62	−1.271	12	0.228
/i/ Modal Pre /i/ Modal Post	154 189	75 73	−1.431	12	0.178
/a/ 8va Pre /a/ 8va Post	243 251	77 79	−0.066	12	0.949
/i/ 8va Pre /i/ 8va Post	223 247	72 93	−0.738	12	0.475
Experimental					
/a/ Modal Pre /a/ Modal Post	159 163	55 52	−0.421	14	0.680
/i/ Modal Pre /i/ Modal Post	171 173	54 62	−0.189	14	0.853
/a/ 8va Pre /a/ 8va Post	265 254	117 77	0.429	14	0.674
/i/ 8va Pre /i/ 8va Post	220 204	104 67	0.778	14	0.450

There were no significant differences between the groups at either testing point and neither group showed significant change across the testing points. The differences between the modal voice and one octave higher recordings are in agreement for the statistics from the whole group of 29 subjects, with mean flow rates through the higher pitched vowels being significantly greater.

A crosstab of percentage of change (Table 5.5) was also carried out, evaluating movement around the mean. Change away from the normal range, one standard deviation on either side of the mean, was considered as deterioration, while change towards the normal range was considered improvement.

Table 5.5 Percentage of the subjects showing change by group.

Group	Deterioration	No Change	Improvement
Control	6	4	3
Experimental	5	4	6

The results shown in Table 5.5 suggest that the Experimental group showed more improvement and less deterioration than the Control group. Analysis, however, indicated that these results were not statistically significant (Pearson Chi-Square Value 4.998, $df = 4$, $p = 0.358$). The Pearson Chi-Square is another less powerful statistical test that is used with this type of comparison for identifying differences.

All data used for the above statistical analysis consisted of the Mean Flow Rate through steady state vowels. Further detail is provided through qualitative assessment of the Aerophone II tracings (see Figures 5.1–5.4), which demonstrate some significant differences in tracing morphology that would not appear when mean flow measures were taken.

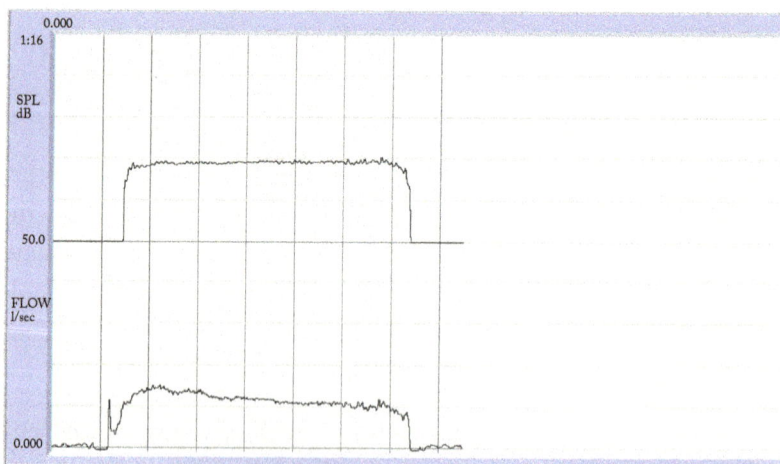

Figure 5.1 Airflow tracing morphology. MFR tracing /a/ 8va from a female subject, showing typical morphology

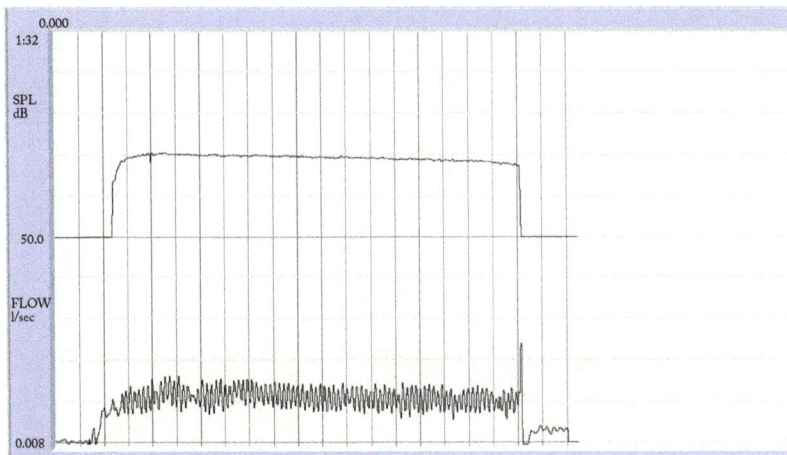

Figure 5.2 Airflow tracing morphology. MRF tracing /a/ 8va from a female subject showing atypical morphology

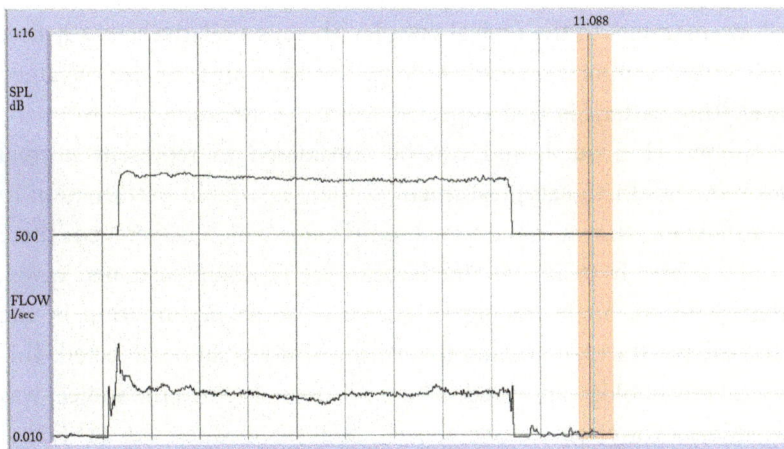

Figure 5.3 Airflow tracing morphology. MFR tracing /a/ 8va from a male subject showing typical morphology

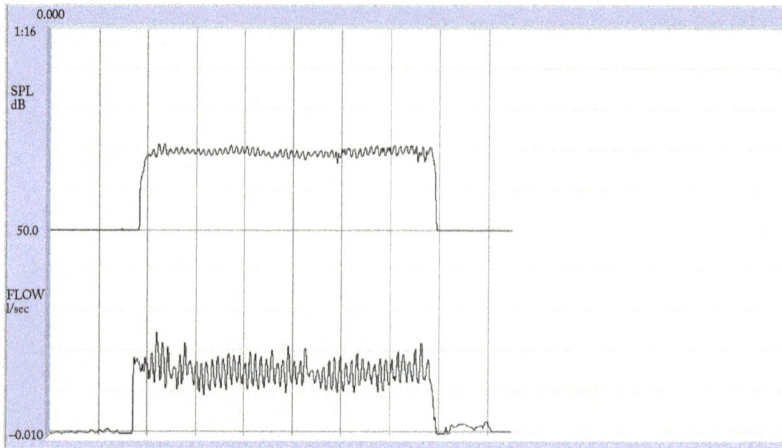

Figure 5.4 Airflow tracing morphology. MFR tracing /a/ 8va from a male subject showing atypical morphology

As these four MFR tracings show, there are two distinct patterns of airflow emerging. In the typical samples, there is a relatively steady flow of air which supports a steady volume level for most of the sustained vowel. This pattern is that expected from the literature and from the Aerophone II manual, and can be considered to represent normal airflow traces. In the atypical tracings, there is a rapid perturbation in the airflow not shown in the actual MFR value which is averaged. There is still a relatively steady volume level in the resultant sustained vowel, although in the male tracing (Figure 5.4) some perturbation in the SPL (volume trace), matching that of the airflow, can be detected. This atypical morphology appeared to be more obvious when the subject was sustaining a vowel one octave above modal pitch, when the MFR was always higher. These atypical tracings were seen in five subjects of the control group at the initial pre-training assessment and in an additional two of the control group at the second post-training assessment (total of seven subjects). There were four subjects from the Experimental group who had these atypical morphologies at the initial assessment, but only one of them still demonstrated the atypical morphology at the second, post-training assessment.

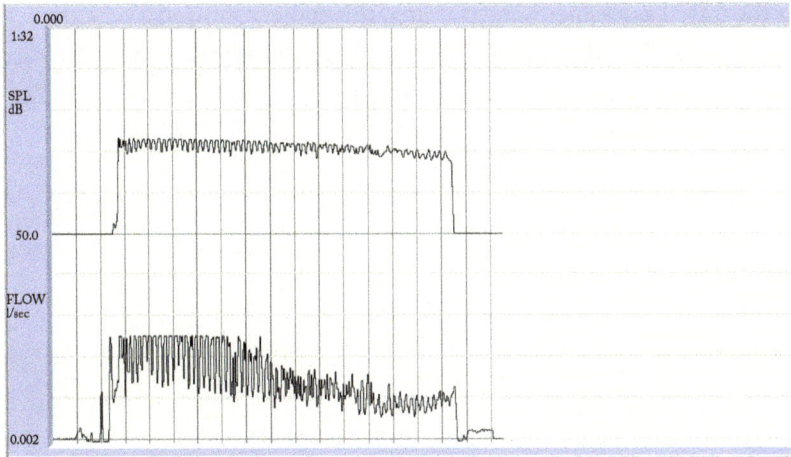

A. Pre-intervention

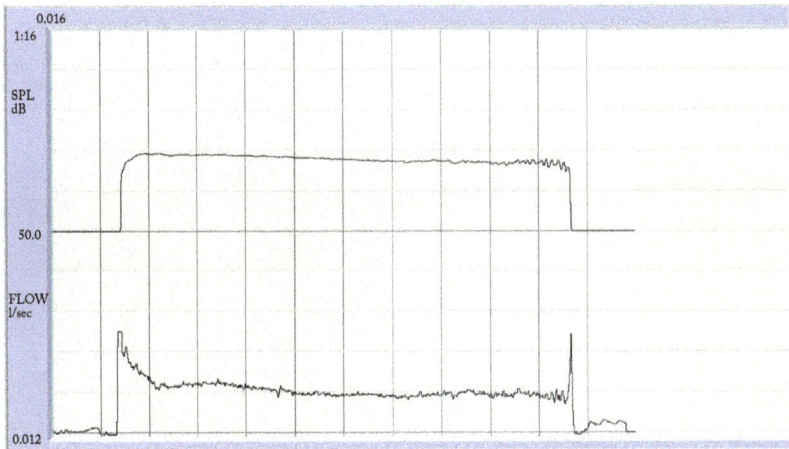

B. Post intervention

Figure 5.5 MFR tracing /a/ 8va from Subject 1 (Experimental group male) showing atypical morphology pre-training (a), but typical morphology in post-training (b)

At the initial assessment pre-training, this subject showed a very atypical pattern of airflow that was also affecting the steadiness of the SPL trace. Post-training with the Accent Method, this subject is now showing a normal pattern, with both steady airflow and steady SPL traces.

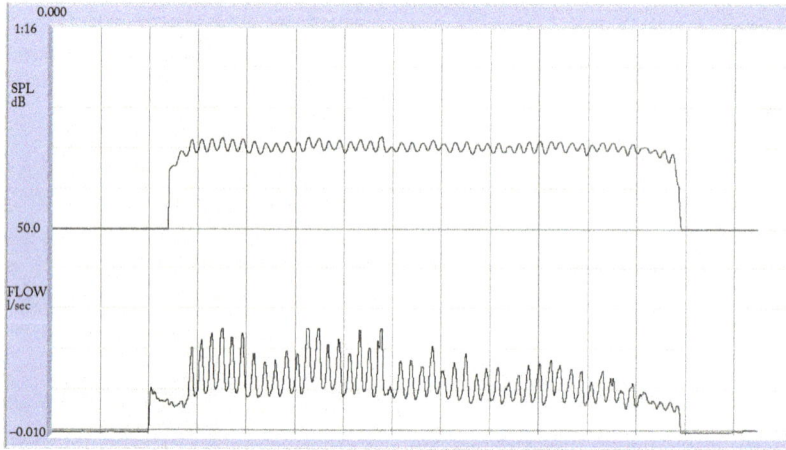

A. Pre-intervention

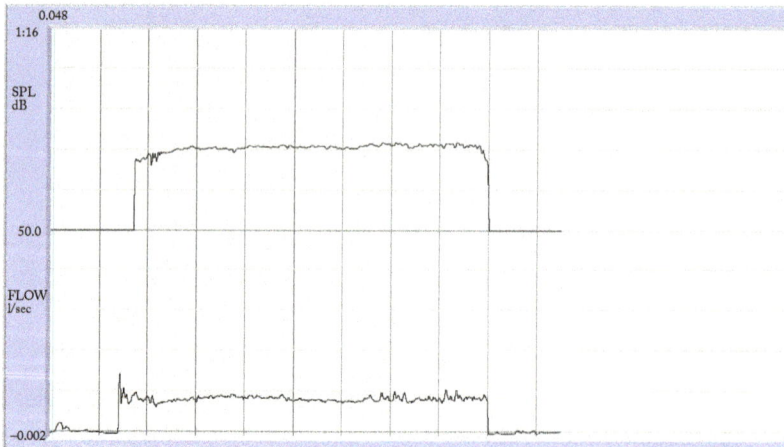

B. Post intervention

Figure 5.6 MRF tracing /a/ 8va from Subject 3 (Experimental group female) showing atypical morphology Pre-training (a), but typical morphology Post-training (b).

Subject 3's airflow traces (Figure 5.6) again show an atypical pattern at the initial assessment but typical airflow and dB SPL patterns at the second assessment following training with the Accent Method. This subject showed a marked fluctuation in the dB SPL trace initially, but this was eliminated in the post-training tracing.

As none of the subjects in the Control group who had atypical patterns at initial assessment changed towards more typical patterns at the second post-training assessment, it appears that training with the Accent Method was instrumental in bringing about change towards a more typical pattern. Two additional subjects from the Control group showed atypical patterns at the post-training session having shown typical patterns initially, but no subjects from the Experimental group changed from a typical to an atypical pattern.

Phonetograms

The results of the phonetograms were averaged to allow easier statistical analysis (Table 5.6). Averaging dynamic ranges and the maximum number of semitones sung allowed the male and female singers, who have different pitch ranges, to be analysed together.

Table 5.6 Average dynamic range in decibels by Control and Experimental groups

Group/Task	M	SD	t	df	Sig (2-tailed)
Cont Pre	21.56	5.90	−1.843	13	0.088
Cont Post	24.40	4.32			
Exp Pre	21.61	6.32	−4.757 ***	14	0.000
Exp Post	28.41	3.45			

Note. Cont = control group, Exp = experimental group, *** = $p < 0.001$. Please note that this is even more significant than $p = 0.01$; it suggests that there is a 99.9% chance that the change is due to the Accent Method.

The Experimental group had a significantly wider dynamic range post-training than at the initial pre-training assessment. On the other hand, the Control group showed no statistically significant differences across the two testing points. This suggests that the training received by the Experimental group was responsible for bringing about change.

The maximum number of semitones was also assessed by group (Table 5.7).

Table 5.7 Maximum number of semitones sung by Control and Experimental groups

Group/Task	*M*	*SD*	*t*	*df*	Sig (2-tailed)
Cont Max S Pre	37.57	3.48	−1.415	13	0.180
Cont Max S Post	39.00	2.03			
Exp Max S Pre	35.73	2.54	−3.437 **	14	0.004
Exp Max S Post	38.73	3.49			

Note. Max S = Maximum number of semitones sung, ** = $p < 0.01$.

These results (Table 5.7) indicate that the experimental group had significantly more semitones in their range post-training than they did initially. There were no significant differences for the control group.

Average dynamic ranges were used in the statistical analysis of the data. This allowed an easy comparison between the two groups, as differences in the number of semitones sung would not affect the outcome. It is also possible to look graphically at the phonetograms that were obtained for each group, presented in Figures 5.7–5.9. Average minima and maxima for each semitone sung were calculated, and male and female singers were combined to provide a single phonetogram based on each group's data.

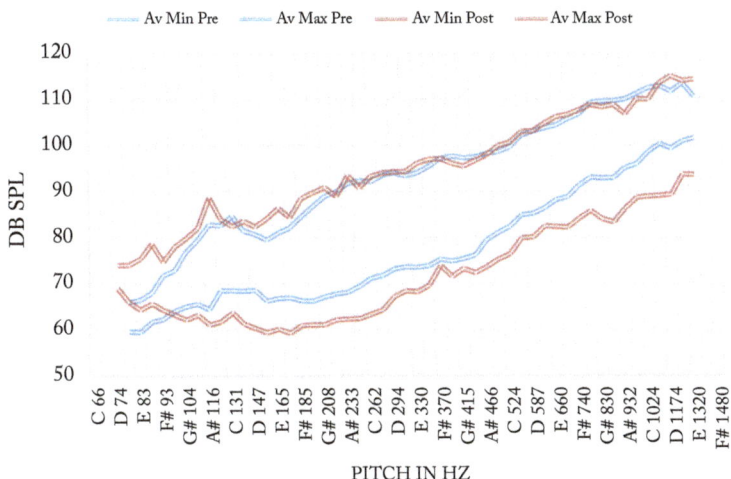

Figure 5.7 Phonetogram for the Control group pre- and post-training

This phonetogram (Figure 5.7) shows that there was some change in the dynamic ranges for the singers in the Control group. These changes were not statistically significant, but they do show some ability to sing more softly at the post-training assessment than was possible initially ($t = -1.843$, $df = 13$ and $p = 0.088$).

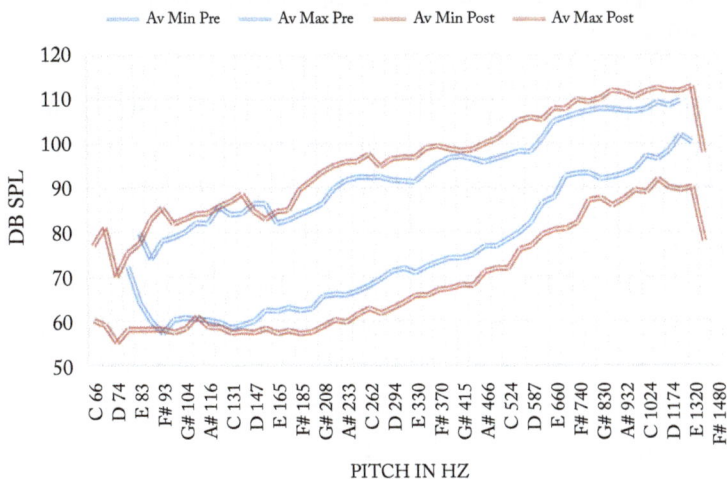

Figure 5.8 Phonetogram for the Experimental group pre- and post-training with Accent Method

The phonetogram in Figure 5.8 shows a clear difference between the pre- and post-training recordings. A highly significant difference was seen in the average dynamic range measures (t = −4.757, df = 14 and p = 0.000.), with the subjects in the Experimental group showing improvement in their ability to sing both softly and loudly. The total number of semitones sung was also significantly greater (t = −3.437, df = 14, p = 0.004).

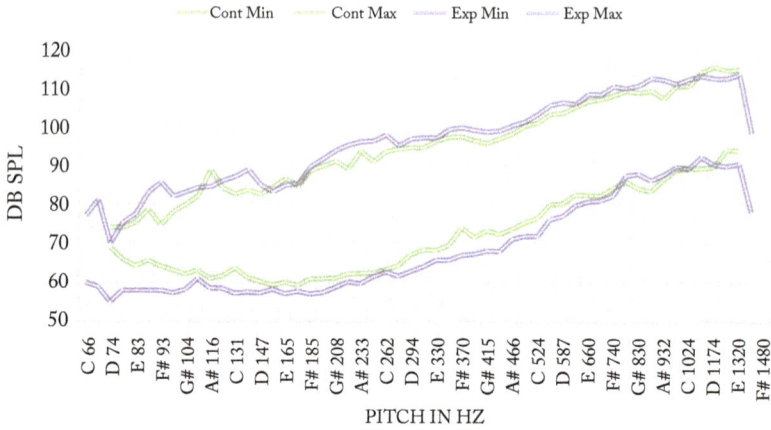

Figure 5.9 Comparison of the Control and Experimental group phonetograms post-training

The phonetogram (Figure 5.9) for the Experimental group is larger overall, with both soft and loud tones showing an advantage. The mean dynamic ranges were statistically significant (t = −2.768, df = 27 and p = 0.01).

There were also considerable variations in the phonetograms of individual singers. No subject's phonetogram was smaller at the post-training assessment than it was initially. The phonetograms shown below (Figures 5.10–5.13) represent the degree of change seen for two male and two female subjects in the Experimental group.

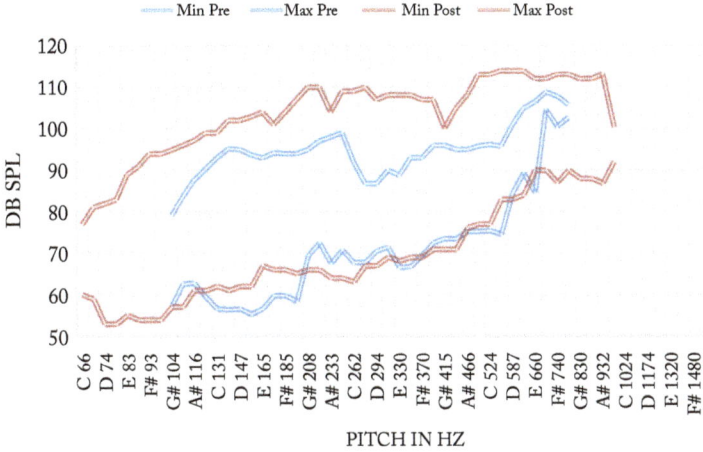

Figure 5.10 Phonetogram of a male subject from the Experimental group showing a large degree of change

The phonetogram for Subject 13 (Figure 5.10) shows an increase in both the dynamic range and in the maximum number of semitones sung. This subject shows a clear advantage for the louder tones throughout the frequency range, with his average dynamic range increasing by 10 dB. An additional eight semitones were available at the lower end of his range, with four more available in his highest register.

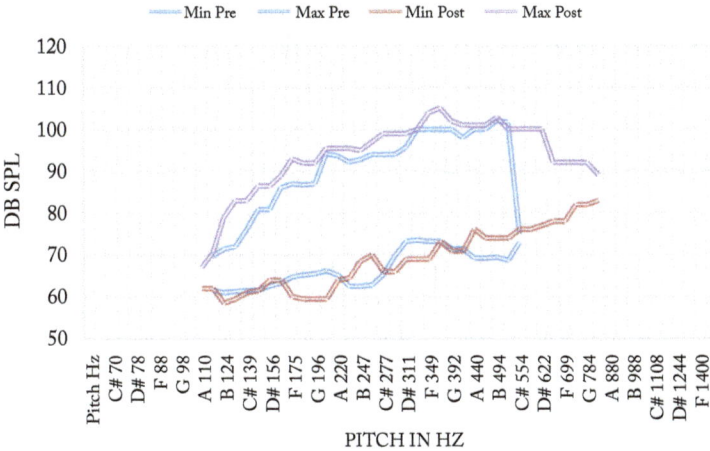

Figure 5.11 Phonetogram of a male subject from the Experimental group showing a lesser degree of change

Subject 10's phonetogram (Figure 5.11) does show improvement between the two testing points, although the difference is not as great as that for subject 13. Subject 10 shows an increase in the average dynamic range of less than 1 dB, but there was an increase of eight semitones in the higher registers.

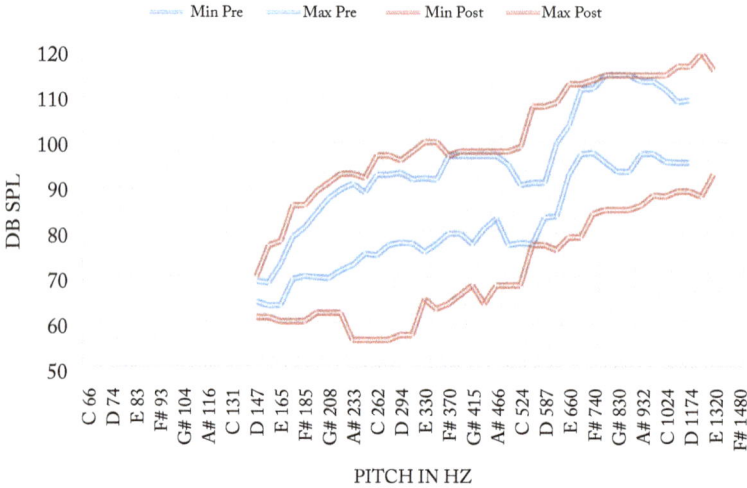

Figure 5.12 Phonetogram of a female subject from the Experimental group showing a large degree of change

Subject 11 again shows a large increase in the dynamic range across the two testing points (Figure 5.12), with an increase in the average dynamic range of 15 dB. Her improvement in the total number of semitones sung was smaller, with only two additional semitones sung.

Subject 6 showed a lesser degree of change. Her phonetogram (Figure 5.13) showed a greater facility for soft singing, which was reflected in an additional 7 dB in the average dynamic range, but she was only able to increase her total semitones sung by one.

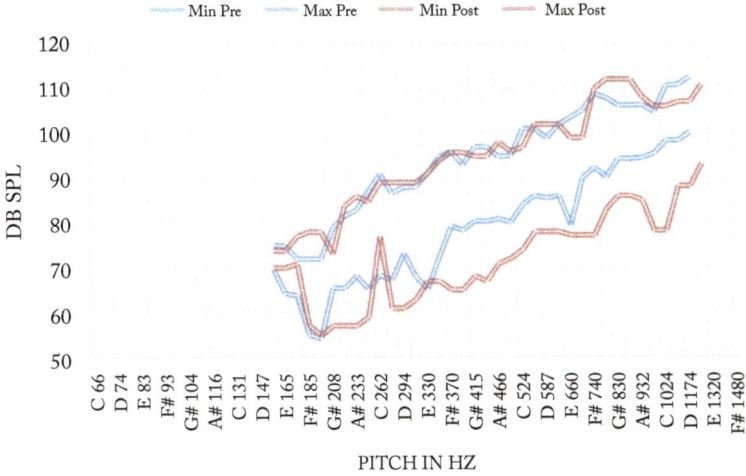

Figure 5.13 Phonetogram of a female subject from the Experimental group showing a lesser degree of change

Perceptual judgments

Perceptual judgment remains one of the most important ways to evaluate voices. This is particularly important when the singing voice is under scrutiny. The opinion of trained judges is considered to be highly valuable for identifying change. Judge preferences were taken into account in this study by giving a value of 1 when the judge preferred the pre-training recording, and a value of 2 if they preferred the post-training recording. The results are shown in Table 5.8.

Table 5.8 Judge's preferences for recording of 'Caro Mio Ben' by group

Group	M	SD	t	df	Sig (2-tailed)
Control	1.41	0.36	-2.624 *	27	0.014
Experimental	1.73	0.29			

Note. * = $p < 0.05$.

These results (Table 5.8) indicate that more of the post-training recordings from the Experimental group were preferred over those pre-training. In the Control group however, a greater number of the pre-training recordings were preferred.

Maximum phonation times

Maximum phonation times (MPT) were recorded by asking the subjects to take a breath and sustain the required vowel for as long as possible, at a comfortable level of loudness. A standard microphone was used for the recording. The results are detailed below in Table 5.9.

Table 5.9 maximum phonation times in seconds via the microphone for recordings /a/ and /i/, with results from paired t-tests assessing difference across the training

Group/Task	*M*	*SD*	*t*	*df*	Sig. (2-tailed)
Control					
/a/ Pre	20.33	6.01	−1.561	13	0.142
/a/ Post	22.22	7.02			
/i/ Pre	23.34	6.86	−0.706	13	0.493
/i/ Post	24.18	6.91			
Experimental					
/a/ Pre	17.94	4.30	−0.255	14	0.803
/a/ Post	18.19	3.91			
/i/ Pre	18.93	4.37	−0.933	14	0.366
/i/ Post	19.63	4.87			

Note. Pre = January (pre-training), Post = March (post-training).

There were no significant differences observed post-training within either the Control or Experimental groups. Both groups showed a slightly longer phonation time post-training, than at the initial assessment, but these differences were not statistically significant. Analysis of the results between groups showed a longer phonation time for the /i/ vowel in the control group at the post-training recording, ($t = 2.058$, $df = 27$, $p = .049$). The difference is very similar to that observed between the two groups pre-training, and suggests that the difference seen on initial assessment has continued to exist.

In conclusion, although there was no improvement in the maximum phonation times or mean airflow measures in the study, there were very significant improvements in the dynamic ranges and airflow tracing morphology that could be attributed to the Accent Method. Trained and experienced judges also preferred the singing of the students who had received the Accent Method training.

6

The Accent Method: the first steps

These first stages in breath management are vital. They encourage 'letting go' of tension in the vocal tract, allowing the breathing muscles to work naturally. Singers and performers often find this stage the most difficult; they seem to think that they always have to 'do' something. If these initial stages have not been established, moving on to the sequence of rhythmic exercises will be somewhat pointless.

We start the exercises on the floor. The advantages of this are:

- Better postural alignment
- The diaphragm has a mechanical advantage for breathing in
- Rib cage is naturally slightly elevated, neck is lengthened, shoulders relaxed
- The respiratory system works naturally in this relaxed position
- The awareness of alignment and breathing is easier
- The floor is the 'support' so there is no 'fighting gravity'

Lie on the floor on your back, knees bent, with the soles of your feet flat on the floor (Figure 6.1). If needed, put a small cushion or book under your head to achieve correct alignment. Place your hands on your abdomen (for most people, thumbs level with the navel and fingers pointing downwards. Those with a 'low slung' navel should place the thumb on the waist, with the fingers resting just above the pubic bone).

If relaxed, you should feel the breath moving your hands gently up and down. There should be very little movement in the upper chest if you are allowing the diaphragm to work naturally. Take time. The more you relax and let go, the easier it becomes.

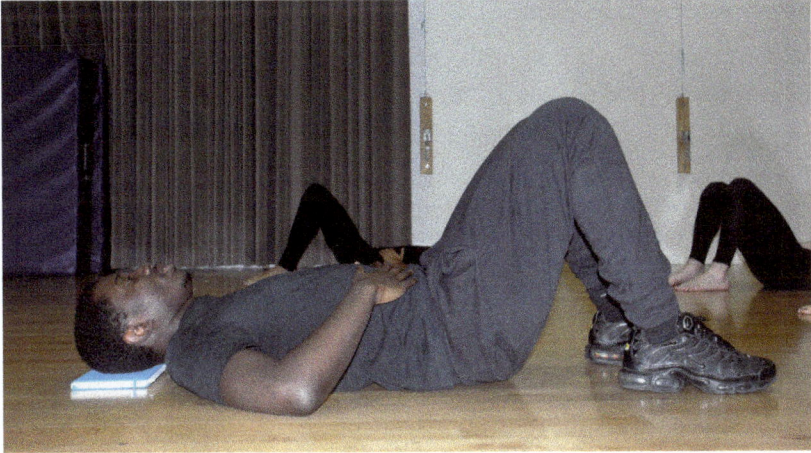

Figure 6.1 Photograph showing the initial position (semi-supine). Note the book placed under the head to ensure comfortable alignment of the neck.

Spend some time breathing in this position. When you feel comfortable and relaxed, you should start to become more aware of your breathing pattern. Generally there are three types:

1. *In – out – in – out (no pause)*

2. *In – hold – out – in – hold - out*

3. *In – out – small pause – in – out – small pause*

Good tidal breathing is pattern three, that is, the sense of a small pause after exhaling. Aim to work in this way.

Once completely comfortable with breathing in this way, the next step is to take the diaphragm under your voluntary control to breathe in.

As explained in Chapter 1, the diaphragm is not completely under our voluntary control, but we can activate it to breathe in. We simply send a message from the brain that we are going to breathe in, and the respiratory system should respond as it did during tidal breathing.

With the hands still in position, you will feel, as the diaphragm descends, the upward movement of the abdominal wall. There will be a corresponding downward movement as the breath is released.

When you feel you can do this easily, move on to the next stage which is to use voiceless fricatives. Fricatives are sounds that are made on a continuous stream of air that passes through a point of constriction. In the exercises we use:

- /s/ the tongue and the alveolar ridge (tooth ridge) as in 'sun'

- /f/ the top teeth and the bottom lip as in 'foot'

- /ʃ/ (sh) the tongue and the hard palate as in 'shoe'

- /θ/ (th) the tongue between the teeth as in 'thumb'.

Take a breath as before but now, as you release the air, gently sigh on one of the fricative sounds. At the beginning, you might find one fricative sound works better than the others, but with practice, you should be able to use all the fricatives equally well. It is important that when making the sounds, the tongue, lips and jaw should be loose. **There should be no attempt to control the length of the out breath.**

Once you can use the voiceless fricatives easily and without tension, move to their voiced equivalents. Modal voice (Mechanism 1, Chest voice) must be used.

- /s/ becomes /z/. /z/ as in 'zoo'.

- /f/ becomes /v/. /v/ as in 'voice'.

- /ʃ/ becomes /ʒ/ (zh). /ʒ/ as in 'measure'.

- /θ/ becomes /ð/. /ð/ as in 'this'.

It is also possible to use : semi-vowel /w/ and the close vowel /y/ (similar to French u, or German ü).

When using voiced sounds, you should aim for 'airy and light'. It is important that there is no unnecessary tension in the vocal tract.

These exercises form the foundation for the rest of the breath and support work. They must be done easily and comfortably before moving to the other positions:

- Side lying
- Sitting
- Standing.

Lying on the side

In this position, the diaphragm has less mechanical advantage for breathing in, so the abdominal wall must relax to allow the diaphragm to move down. Also, less help is provided by gravity on the out breath, so there needs to be a slightly more deliberate movement of the abdominal wall inwards and upwards. Repeat all the above exercises in this positon. When the exercises are done easily and comfortably in this position, move to sitting.

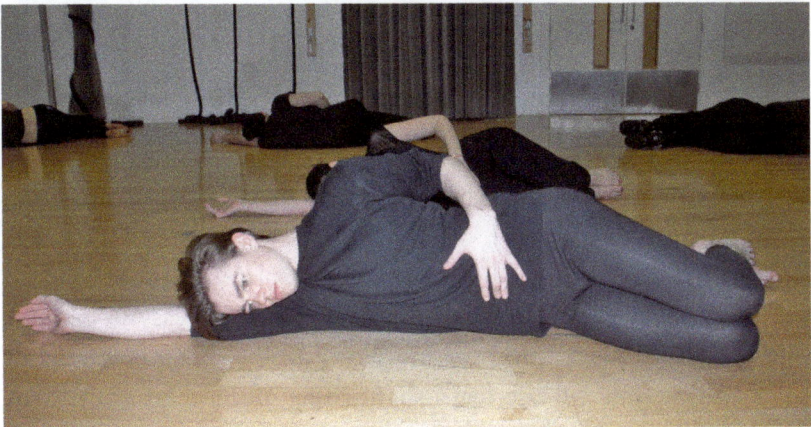

Figure 6.2 Photograph showing the side lying position. Alignment of the neck remains important and books can still be used if required.

Sitting

It can sometimes be difficult to maintain abdominal–diaphragmatic breathing when moving from the floor to a chair. Good postural alignment in the chair will make it easier to maintain the breathing pattern.

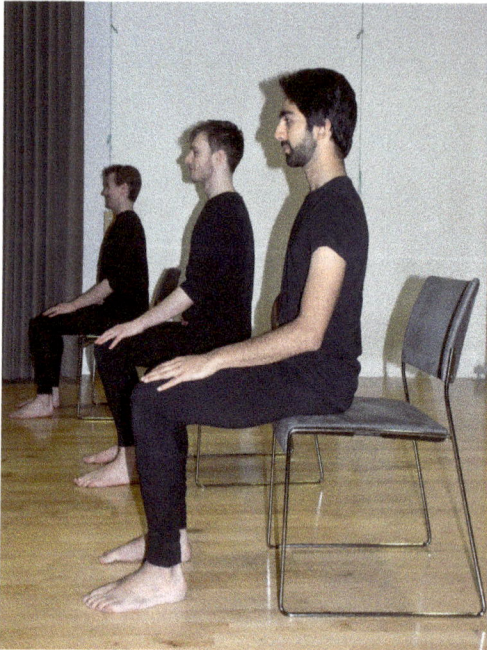

Figure 6.3 Photograph showing the sitting position. Again, alignment is vital. Many chairs are unsuitable as they would distort the pelvic and lower back position (as in this example), so it is often necessary to move the student further forward in the chair, as shown here.

Keeping one hand on the abdomen as before, place the other hand on the upper chest. With the hands in this position it is easy to monitor your breathing. You will feel the movement in the abdominal wall but on exhalation, you will also feel a **slight** rising of the chest as the air is expelled. On the next in breath, the chest will return to a **slightly** lower position.

Practise all the sounds as before (both voiceless and voiced). Once you can do this easily and comfortably, move to the standing position.

Standing

It is important to check postural alignment as this is essential for good breathing. Practise all the sounds as before, and use the hands to monitor breathing.

Remember: in any position, there should be no unnecessary tension in the tongue, lips, jaw and throat. No attempt should be made to extend the out breath. Sigh easily.

Support

For singing, we need to add 'support'. Support is muscular energy that is used to manipulate the respiratory system in order to maintain the appropriate balance of air pressure and airflow. It is flexible, dynamic and ever-changing throughout the musical phrase. Support is **not** tension or rigidity. The exercises so far have not used support; they have been working on airflow and release of tension. This is to ensure that the vocal tract is free and that the throat has no unnecessary muscular tension, i.e. open throat.

With the first stage of the exercises in place, we can now introduce support. Some experienced singers find that they can 'hook back' into their support quite naturally. Others, and less well experienced singers, may need more direct work to access the appropriate muscular energy. Here, we underline the importance of the vocal tract being free of tension: otherwise the throat will not remain open when we add support.

A good way of feeling the muscular energy involved in support is to put one hand on the front of the stomach, as before, and the other hand in the soft tissue just above the hip bone (the side support junction or waistband support). Now cough (gently!), groan, laugh (it's not that funny!) or 'whoop' like a monkey ('oo, oo, oo'). These are all examples of primal sounds. There is an excellent explanation of the neurological basis of primal sound and its uses in singing in Janice Chapman's book, *Singing and teaching singing: A holistic approach to classical voice.*

Adding this support to the exercises

One of the easiest ways to begin to feel the support is to lie on the floor on your side. In this position, the muscular energy needed can be felt on the out breath as the abdomen is engaged more vigorously.

Repeat the fricative exercises with a hand placed on the abdomen. The movement will need to be more vigorous as the abdomen travels inwards and upwards. Now repeat the exercises, but with a hand on the side support junction so that the muscular energy is clearly felt. These exercises help develop the strength of the connection to the support. They raise awareness of the support and are an important intermediate stage. However, the movement of the abdominal wall becomes more subtle as the system is more highly developed and trained.

These support muscles can, however, be turned on at will without using breath. Try doing this. Engage them but don't breathe. Notice how tense and tight the vocal tract is, and how rigid the front of the abdomen becomes. Now make a primal sound which has moving breath. You will feel the same muscular energy but no vocal tract tension, and the abdominal wall remains flexible.

Only use these support muscles for breathing out. Engaging them to breathe in is counterproductive. The vocal tract will become tense, making it more difficult to use good airflow and support on the out-breath. Try it. Notice how tense and tight the upper chest and vocal tract become. When you try to make voiced fricatives, you will feel the tension created on the out-breath.

All the above exercises should be repeated while both sitting and standing. Doing some negative practice, contrasted with correct practice, will help raise awareness of the feeling of appropriate muscular energy.

Once you are off the floor gravity comes into play. The support muscles are now doing 'double duty'. They are not only supporting the out-breath but also, maintaining good postural alignment. Therefore, there may be a perceived reduction in the feeling when they are activated for breathing.

Hands-on monitoring is a powerful and useful tool as it gives the teacher immediate feedback from the student. It also helps the student to feel the correct model from the teacher. It is important to ask, and gain, the student's permission before using any hands-on monitoring. A good way to do this is for the teacher to place the back of his hand on the student's abdomen; the student then covers the teacher's hand with his own. The student can also place the back of his hand on the teacher's abdomen with the teacher then covering the student's hand with his own.

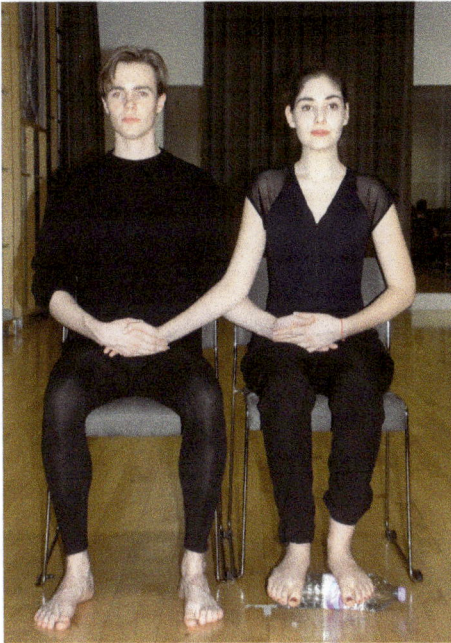

Figure 6.4 Photograph showing the hands in the correct position for monitoring the flexibility of the abdominal wall. Note the use of the water bottle to aid correct alignment. Without this prop under the feet, the leg and pelvic position would not have been appropriate as the chair was too high. Although you can use whatever is to hand (as we have done!) books are very useful.

When practising, use all the sounds mentioned above, in any order, mixing voiceless and voiced. Always start with airflow alone, with no support added, to ensure that the vocal tract remains free and relaxed. Once again, only move on to using support when (guess what!) these exercises become easy and comfortable. Regular practice is essential. Aim for at least 20 minutes each day, which can be split into multiple practice sessions - 'little and often'.

7

The first accent bounce

Now we introduce the first 'bounce' of the abdomen. This gives us:

- Our first accent

- Flexibility of the abdominal wall

- Strength in the abdominal muscles (multiple repetitions build endurance as well!).

Positioning

Start this lying on the side. Before we go to the first accent bounce, we need to find 'tummy neutral'. When working one-to-one, it is easier to get this concept across by monitoring. However, in a group situation it can be more difficult. To recognise 'tummy neutral', exhale all of your available air, then release the tummy but don't actively breathe in. If you are relaxed, some air will go in. Try doing this a couple of times. Once you are familiar with this position, you are ready to go on to the first accent bounce.

We start in a fairly easy 2/4 rhythm. Make sure the air flows continuously but the tummy releases towards neutral between the beats. This gives us our accent. The adjustment of the airflow occurs because of the action of the abdominal muscles, not the larynx. Any adjustment in the larynx happens naturally through this airflow and not by active work in the vocal tract.

First rhythmic pattern.

Our first rhythmic pattern is shown below with the Teacher starting and the Student following:

1st Accent Bounce

Make sure the up-beat is gentle and unaccented.

If you are working on your own, follow one line only, don't 'fill in' the rhythms on the other line. Use all of the fricative sounds. Once easy and comfortable you can start to check for support. If necessary, you can be a bit more vigorous to connect to the support.

As with the first stage, these exercises should be repeated while sitting and standing. Remember our practice mantra: easy and comfortable, little and often.

Adding movement

Once you can do all these exercises easily, you are ready to add whole body movement. The first movement is a swaying motion. Adding this movement has a number of advantages:

- It prevents 'locking' of the body while breathing
- It encourages the correct movement of the abdominal wall

- It allows the singer to experience new breathing patterns while engaged in another motor activity. This helps with the motor learning of the breathing

- It encourages the breathing and support to work, whatever the physical demands of the performance.

Ideally, this swaying should be done in pairs, standing side by side rather like skaters or dancers (corps de ballet!), one foot in front of the other (Figure 7.1). This can be done alone, although you may like to place one hand on the back of a chair as support. Begin swaying forwards and backwards. As you go forward, release the abdomen to breathe in and then, as you go back, feel the abdominal wall moving backwards as you breathe out. Next, increase the swaying movement, making sure that the hips remain flexible, not tight, during each sway. As you sway forward, bend the front knee and release the back leg, allowing the pelvis to move naturally slightly forward and under.

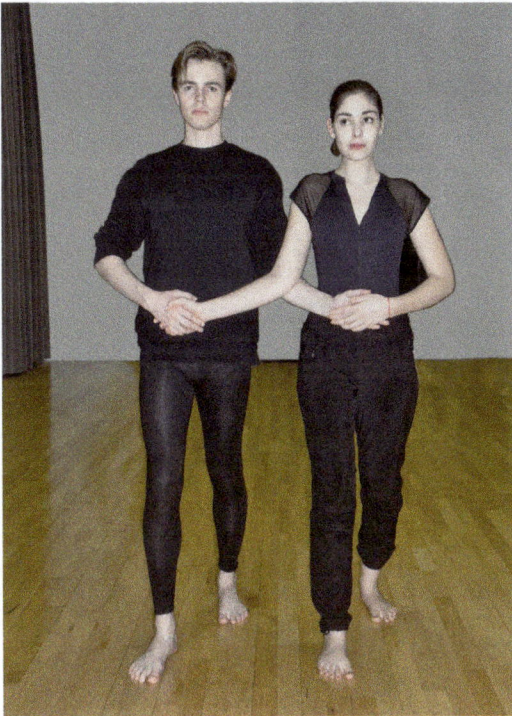

Figure 7.1 Photograph showing the side-by-side swaying position with the hands monitoring abdominal movement.

Perform this swaying movement a few times just using your tidal breathing. Once easy and comfortable (have you noticed it again?), add the fricative sounds, building up to the first accent bounce. After about 20 repetitions (use all of the fricative sounds singly and with the first bounce), change the front foot and repeat. It is rather like a conversation between the teacher and the student.

In a variation of the swaying exercise the teacher and student face each other but in this case, the out-breaths alternate immediately (teacher then student). This is particularly useful if a student tends to hold his breath. All the fricative sounds can be used singly and with the first bounce.

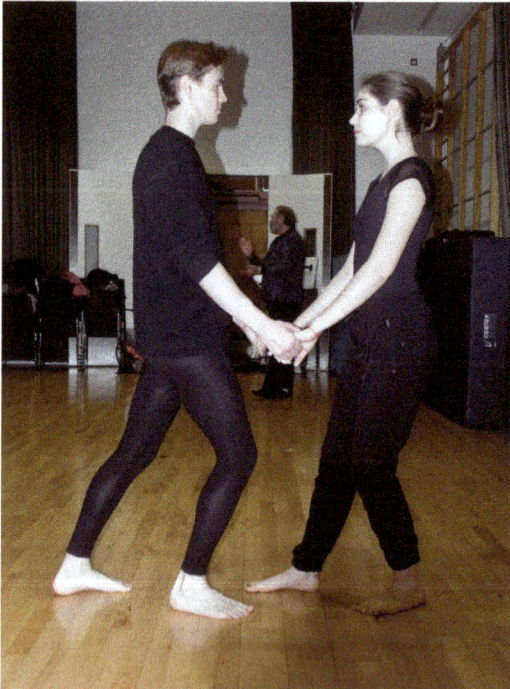

Figure 7.2 Photograph showing the face-to-face swaying position.

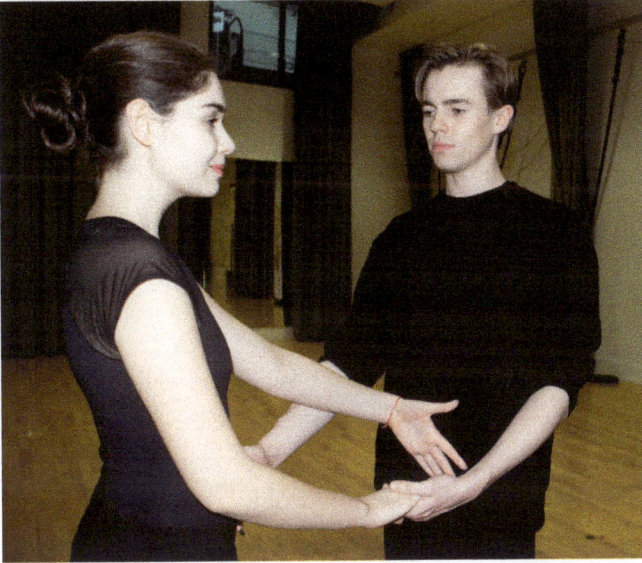

Figure 7.3 Photograph showing the face-to-face swaying positon, with monitoring.

The first accent bounce provides the necessary accent of the airflow and promotes the flexibility of the abdominal wall (tummy). The use of the swaying helps to provide multiple repetitions to encourage strength, endurance and motor learning, as well as to make certain that the hips and knees remain relaxed and free.

8

Rhythmic patterns

Once the initial stages (First Steps and First Bounce) are well established, we move on to rhythmic patterns. We continue to use the conversational concept: the teacher models, the student copies. If done properly, these exercises gradually build up the strength, flexibility and endurance of the abdominal muscles. The rhythmic patterns also enable the singer to be aware of the important relationships between air pressure, airflow and phonation. They help the singer in the development of appropriate co-ordination of breath and voice.

We divide the rhythmic patterns into three groups:

- 3/4 Rhythms

- 4/4 Rhythms

- Complex Rhythms.

3/4 Rhythms

In the original version of the Accent Method, this is known as Tempo 1 Largo. Kirsten Thyme-Frøkjær states that this is the most important voice exercise in the whole system. The speed is reasonably slow and should be based around the student's tidal breathing pattern. A metronome marking of approximately 58 beats per minute (BPM) seems to work well for most people. It is worth remembering that children and the elderly tend to breathe more quickly, so the speed should be altered accordingly.

It is in these rhythmic patterns that a drum is traditionally used. This can be particularly useful when working in groups, as it keeps the group together. When working with individuals, a small hand-held drum can also be used, but it is not vital for work with singers.

We usually introduce the patterns in the seated position first. However, when working with groups, we have found that it is often easier to establish these patterns in the side-lying position initially. When close individual monitoring is not possible, experience has shown that some variations to the usual approach are useful to minimise confusions.

All of the patterns start with a quaver up-beat. The student breathes, in time, on the last beat of the teacher's bar, ready for their own quaver up-beat.

Pattern 1: minim

Pattern 2

In performing this pattern, we are aiming for equal length and strength in both of the accented pulses. For this to work efficiently, a release towards neutral is necessary between the accented pulses.

127

In this variation of Pattern 2, the second accented beat is tied over to a quaver. While the lengths of the two pulses now vary, we still want the strengths of the pulses to remain equal.

Pattern 3

In this pattern, there is not time for a full release to neutral on the quavers, but a small release towards neutral is still necessary. This is important to discourage tightness or tension.

Work through the above patterns at least once with all the fricatives, unvoiced and voiced. The order of the patterns and fricatives can then be varied as desired. Check that the support muscles are responding appropriately to the accented pulses.

Once these patterns can be achieved easily and comfortably in the seated position, move to standing and repeat. Remember that once you are standing, the support muscles are also contributing to your postural alignment.

4/4 Rhythms

In the original version of the Accent Method these are known as Tempo 2 Andante. The extra beat in the 4/4 patterns not only increases the length of the phrase but also, allows for more rhythmic variations. The speed is slightly faster. We find that a metronome setting of approximately 68 BPM works well. Once again, all the upbeats are quavers, with the student breathing on the last beat of the teacher's bar, ready for their own quaver upbeat.

There are six patterns in this group. The patterns are practised in the same conversational way between teacher and student as in the 3/4 rhythms.

These patterns are introduced when either sitting or standing. By this stage, we find it is not always necessary to work through each pattern with all the fricatives. This allows for more flexibility in practice. However, it is important that all patterns and all fricatives are covered at some point.

Gentle reminder! Please continue to monitor the flexibility of the abdominal wall and the connection to the support muscles. Sometimes, with these more complex rhythms, it is possible to become more tight or rigid. The goal is still to release towards neutral between the accented pulses.

Most of our work with singers uses these 4/4 patterns. Through multiple repetitions at this level, singers gain strength, flexibility and endurance of the respiratory system. Remember 'little and often' still applies!

Body and arm movements can be added to any of the 3/4 or 4/4 patterns, although they were originally designed to help free the body. Singers gain an added benefit as it helps integrate the new breathing and support mechanism into the movement required for stage work. Some of the movements are detailed in Chapter 10 as part of the 10-week group programme, but feel free to be inventive.

Complex rhythms

In the original version of the Accent Method this is known as Tempo 3 Allegro. These patterns were relatively quick, up to 120 BPM. It is difficult to feel any sense of release at this speed when using only fricatives. This can lead to some tightening and rigidity in the abdominal wall. We prefer to set a slower speed, with complex one bar patterns, at approximately 80 BPM. In the two bar patterns we aim for approximately 92 BPM. Once we move from fricatives into syllables or vowel babble, faster speeds are possible.

s   s   s   s   s   s   s——→

s   s s s s   s   s——→

s   s   s   s s s s——→

s   s   s   s s s s——→

s   s s s s s s s s s——→

2 bar patterns

These are the patterns we use most often , but there are many possible variations. If you want to, why not give your rhythmic imagination free rein.

As always it is important to practice 'little and often', avoiding tension or rigidity in the abdomen or indeed, the whole body.

131

9

Exercises into singing

One of the most commonly asked questions when working on the Accent Method with singers is "but how does this transfer into my singing?" Over time, with regular practice the breathing patterns become second nature in both the speaking and singing voice. However, we can speed up the integration into the singing voice with specific exercises. Some of these exercises will be familiar to many singers but for our purpose, the focus will be principally on airflow and support.

Students will vary in the rate at which they progress but as a rule of thumb, singing exercises should not be started until the 3/4 patterns are easy and comfortable. This is to give time for the new breathing pattern to be established, minimising the chance of confusion with any earlier breathing patterns they may have had.

As these exercises are primarily concerned with airflow they are suitable for all students, regardless of age or stage of development.

1. Start with a fricative in the speaking voice. Then, taking a pitch between A3 and E4 for women and children and C3 to G3 for men, sing the fricative. The goal is to maintain the balance between muscle and breath energy. Singers often need to be told to switch off their aesthetic button rather than try to make a beautiful sound. The exercise can be repeated at a number of pitches within this range, and on a variety of voiced fricatives. It should feel easy.

2. "Candles and Lilos". Initially performed using a breathy /w/ sound, this exercise can be done with all the voiced fricatives. The two short

accentuations are like blowing out a candle and the five-note pattern like inflating a small lilo in one continuous out-breath. The pitch for this exercise is all within M1 (modal voice).

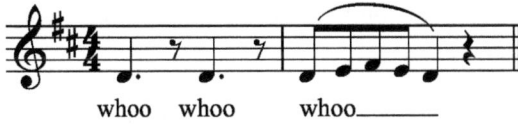

whoo   whoo   whoo_____

3. Fricative Glide over a 5th. This can be done with any fricative, and /ð/ is particularly useful for counteracting tongue root tension! Please see the table in chapter 6 if you are unsure of the sounds represented by the phonetic symbols.

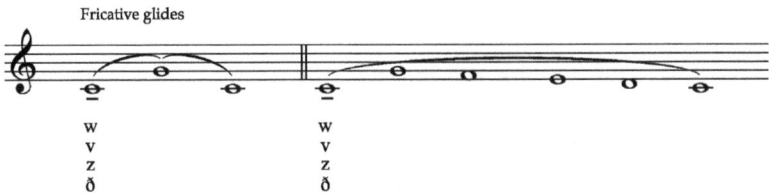

Fricative glides

w   w
v   v
z   z
ð   ð

These can be done throughout a singer's entire range, remembering our 'easy and comfortable' mantra. The emphasis is still on airflow rather than support.

Exercises for airflow and support suitable for all ages and stages of development

1. Bouncing down and up over a 5th. This is done with any voiced fricative or semi-occluded vocal tract sound. Rolled /r/ or the lip trill can be particularly helpful at higher pitches. This exercise is initially carried out in B-flat major for the lower voices and D major for the highervoices. With practice it can be done throughout the compass of the voice. The singer should feel the support muscles engage on each of the downward notes. The support and airflow continue through the run up and down.

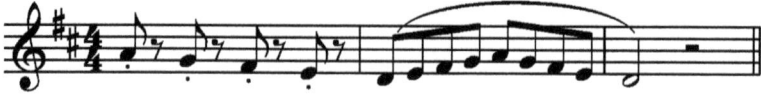

2. Bouncing down and up over the 9th. This is carried out in a similar fashion to the previous exercise.

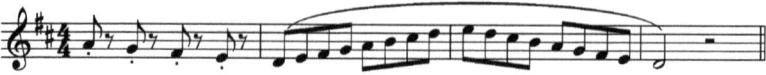

3. Rolled /r/ or lip trill over the 9th scale. If there is a significant degree of tongue root tension on either of these sounds, the floppy rolled /r/ (tongue hanging out with the air flowing continuously, rather like a floppy loose raspberry) can be used. These exercises can be taken throughout the range of the voice. The singer should feel the support muscles engage with the onset of the sound and should continue throughout the entire musical phrase.

If students have difficulty connecting to their support muscles when they move into singing, it helps to adjust their posture for a short time. You can use postural tricks such as:

• Monkey position – maintaining alignment of the head and neck, bend the knees and tilt forward from the hips.

• Elbows to the knees – sitting in a chair, keeping the back straight, head in alignment, tilt forward from the hips and rest the elbows on the knees.

• Leaning on the grand piano – knees bent, fold the arms, lean forward onto the piano, maintaining alignment of the head and neck. For those who do not have a grand piano a sturdy chair back can be used!

• Wall sitting – maintaining alignment of the head and neck, align the back and shoulders against the wall, with knees bent as in a sitting position.

Remember that when it is right, support feels suspiciously easy. However, hands placed on the muscle junctions will let you feel the appropriate activity. When singing, the abdomen does not bounce as it did for the exercises. The singer should feel the abdominal wall moving slowly but surely inwards.

We suggest that the following exercises are best used for the more developed singer. We caution against using them for unchanged voices. When the larynx is not fully developed there is a danger that the weightiness of the exercises can recruit too much additional muscle tension in the vocal tract.

1. Calling out. Using a reflexive cry, "Hey!", "What!", "Wow!" feel the support engage. Then repeat these on a few pitches moving downward, still calling rather than "singing". The support muscles are engaged each time you call. These can then be sung moving down a five note scale. This can be taken up to A flat major so that the starting note is E flat 5 for women and the octave lower for men.

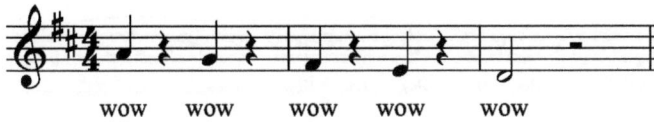

wow   wow   wow   wow   wow

2. Hey Ha exercise – This is carefully set out in Janice Chapman's book *Singing and teaching singing – A holistic approach to classical voice.*

All the above exercises are particularly designed to help singers connect to their breathing and support. Over time this connection should become second nature. However, any technical exercise can be used to remind the singer of good airflow and support.

The "Hey-ha" exercise

1. Stand well with hands firmly on waistband muscle junctions.

2. Shout "hey" as if to someone across the street, noticing the bulking up of the muscle junction.

3. Sing "Hey-ha" on single pitch, repeated through a comfortable range, checking for full release between each sung note (i.e. the waistband muscles must disengage).

Hey,   Ha,   Hey,   Ha,   Hey

4. Sing up a major scale "hey" (release), "ha" (release). On the ascending scale, each note of the scale activates the support and each rest indicates the release. On the descending scale, the support is maintained under a single "hah" with the release after the end of phonation.

Hey, Ha, Hey, Ha, Hey, Ha, Hey, Ha

Note: The impulse for the engagement of this muscle junction must be the movement of the belly wall toward the spine, as occurs in primal sound making (see Chapman, 2006, chapter 4). It is possible for singers to consciously 'flare' the waistband muscles, but this can become a counterproductive manoeuvre if it is not allied to breath flow.

5. Repeat step 4, but add as many scales on the legato "ha" as the performer has air for. This trains the system to achieve more strength and flexibility.

"Hey-ha" exercise from *Singing and teaching singing: A holistic approach to classical voice* by Janice Chapman. Reproduced by kind permission of Plural Publishing, Inc., San Diego.

10

A 10 week course for group teaching

This chapter sets out the Accent Method programme that was taught to the experimental group as part of the research project, the results of which are presented in Chapter 5. Groups of six to 10 students are ideal. When working with a larger group it is better to have two teachers. It is important to be able to monitor the students effectively. This programme is based on over 10 years' experience of teaching groups.

In most cases group teaching is effective. However, one-to-one instruction is sometimes needed to tailor a programme to the student's specific needs and allow for closer monitoring.

Session one

- Accent Method. The First Steps as set out in Chapter 6.

- It is vital when working with groups that good tidal breathing and easy, comfortable airflow with the fricative sounds is established. At this stage support is not added to the airflow exercises.

- Students should wear comfortable clothes that allow for movement and, preferably, be without shoes.

Session two

- Work from the previous session is revised and practised. The majority of this session is spent on the floor to encourage the correct breathing patterns and to promote good postural alignment.

- In this session support can be introduced into the exercises (See Chapter 6).

Session three

- Work from the previous two sessions is revised and practised.

- The first accent bounce (the initial accentuation) is introduced as set out in Chapter 7.

Session four

- As before, revision and practice of the work from previous sessions is carried out.

- The first of the rhythmic patterns is introduced. These are the 3/4 rhythms set out in Chapter 8.

- Arm movements are added for the first time.

- Students stand with feet a shoulder/hip width apart, with good postural alignment and knees unlocked. A pattern of three beats with one beat of rest is used. The students SPLAT the in-breath and then three equal out-breaths are used. The airflow should continue between the accents as in the 3/4 patterns; /s/ is usually used until the patterns are established. Once the abdominal movements and the breath flow are working well, the arms are added. The arm movement is a gesture from the centre of the body outwards so that the movement finishes palms up: right arm out then back to centre, left arm out then back to centre, Both arms out. Repeat as required.

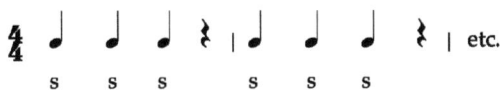

Movement pattern 1

- All the sounds are practised with arm movements.

- The 'cool down' phase is introduced for the first time. Students sit for this: first 3/4 patterns, then the first Accent bounce, finishing with sighing of the air.

- Students are asked to practise their Accent exercises for 15 to 20 minutes daily; they can be broken into smaller chunks, "little and often!"

Session five

- A fairly quick revision of the floor position, sighing of air and the first accent bounce is carried out. The 3/4 patterns are revised in the side lying position on the floor.

- Swaying, both side-by-side and face-to–face, are practised with single sounds and with the first Accent Bounce (See Chapter 7).

- Movement, as before, is practised and then a stepping on the spot leg movement is added. Right arm, right leg, then left arm, left leg, and finally both arms, right leg. There is then one beat of rest before the sequence is started again. This is carried out with all the sounds. The students are then asked to move around the room in a right-left-stop pattern.

- These stepping and arm movements challenge the students' core stability. They help ensure that breath management is not disturbed or altered by the addition of movement. This is essential for stage work.

- The students then move to the chair where 3/4 patterns are practised.

- 4/4 rhythms are introduced (see Chapter 8 - 4/4 patterns).

Study Patterns 4/4

- 3/4 and 4/4 patterns are then practised standing up.

- Cool down again occurs in the chair from 4/4 backwards through 3/4 and first Accent Bounce to sighing of air.

- Connection (breath to voice)to singing exercises are started. Students practise voiced fricatives, and fricatives releasing to vowels, on single pitches in a comfortable middle part of the voice. Correct connection to the support junctions are described and monitored both by the teacher and the student.

- Students are asked to practise the exercises for 15 to 20 minutes daily remebering that they can be broken into smaller chunks, "little and often!"

Session six

- A brief revision of floor positions, sighing of air and first Accent Bounce arecarried out; 3/4 patterns are also practised in the side lying position on the floor.

- Swaying, side-by-side and face-to-face, is performed with single sounds and first Accent Bounce patterns.

- Arm and leg movements in 4/4 are practised, using all of the fricatives and /w and y/.

- A 6/4 pattern for movement is introduced consisting of four beats of vocalization and two bars of rest.

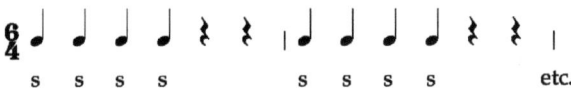

Study Patterns 6/4 Movement

- Once this pattern of breathing is established, marching on the spot (right, left, right, left etc.) is introduced. The feet continue throughout the entire six beats. The breathing and therefore the abdominals have two beats of rest.

- Once the movement of the feet is well established, add swinging arms bent at the elbow. All of the sounds are practised while marching on the spot. Finally, move around the room.

- The students then practise all the patterns learnt thus far, sitting in a chair.

- No new patterns are introduced in this session but vowel sounds other than /y/ are used for the first time. Vowels are released from a voiced fricative on the last beat of the 3/4 patterns. Support and airflow through the vowel should be the same as through the voiced fricative alone. This can be easily monitored at the support junctions by both teacher and student. The five cardinal Italian vowels (/i ,e, a, ɔ and u/)are used, released from the voiced fricatives /z, ʒ, v and ð/ and the semi-vowel /w/. Once these are well established, vowels and diphthongs from other languages, including English, are used.

z z zah
z z zee

z z z zah
etc.

z zah ⟶

Study Patterns ¾ Release onto Vowels

- 4/4 patterns are practised with the fricatives and with /w and y/. Both 3/4 and 4/4 rhythms are practised sitting and standing.

- Cool down again takes place in the chair, moving through 4/4, to 3/4 with vowel release, to 3/4 with fricatives, first Accent Bounce and finally, sighing air.

- Connection to singing continues with the use of fricative-vowel syllables on single pitches and over a pentatonic scale. Students are encouraged to feel the activity at the abdominal support junctions as the abdominal wall continues to move inwards. The 'Hey-Ha' exercise in Janice Chapman's book (see Chapter 9) is introduced.

The "Hey-ha" exercise

1. Stand well with hands firmly on waistband muscle junctions.

2. Shout "hey" as if to someone across the street, noticing the bulking up of the muscle junction.

3. Sing "Hey-ha" on single pitch, repeated through a comfortable range, checking for full release between each sung note (i.e. the waistband muscles must disengage).

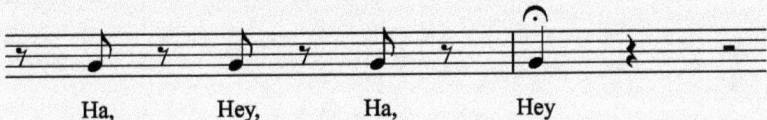

Ha,   Hey,   Ha,   Hey

"Hey-ha" exercise from *Singing and teaching singing: A holistic approach to classical voice* by Janice Chapman. Reproduced by kind permission of Plural Publishing, Inc., San Diego.

- Students are once more asked to practise their Accent exercises for 15 to 20 minutes daily, remembering that they can be broken into smaller chunks, 'little and often!'

Session seven

- Revision of the early sessions is now quite brief, but a few minutes are spent on the floor revising first Accent bounce and 3/4 patterns in the semi-supine and side lying positions.

- Work continues with swaying and arm and body movements as described above, before moving to the chair for pattern practice.

- 3/4 patterns are practised with fricative babble using any combination of voiced fricative consonant or /w/ plus the vowel.

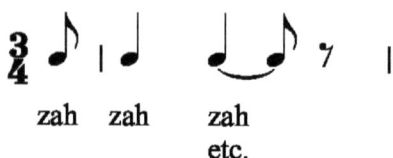

zah   zah   zah
etc.

Study Patterns 3/4 Fricative Babble

- 4/4 patterns are practised with release onto vowels from a voiced fricative (as described above for the 3/4 patterns).

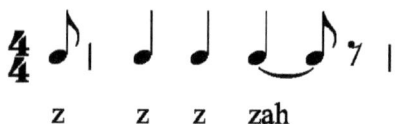

z   z   z   zah

Study Patterns 4/4 Release to Vowels

- The final tempo, Complex Rhythms (Chapter 8- Complex Rhythms), is introduced with fricatives and the sounds /w/ and /y/.

Study patterns complex rhythms

- This is practised in the chair and once established, in a standing position.

- Marching is practised at two speeds, around 65 beats per minute and around 75 beats per minute.

- Cool down again occurs in a sitting position, moving backwards from complex rhythms to sighing of air on fricatives.

- Connection to singing now uses syllables over the whole octave. Glides on fricatives are introduced to encourage connection to the low support muscles. Semi-occluded vocal tract tasks, such as rolled /r/, are introduced (please see exercises described in Chapter 9)

Sing up a major scale "hey" (release), "ha" (release). On the ascending scale, each note of the scale activates the support and each rest indicates the release. On the descending scale, the support is maintained under a single "hah" with the release after the end of phonation.

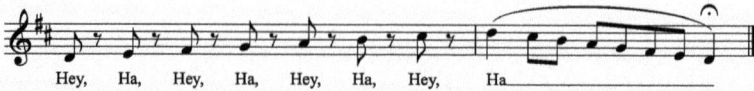

Hey,   Ha,   Hey,   Ha,   Hey,   Ha,   Hey,   Ha

Once again, students are asked to practise their Accent exercises, which can be broken into smaller chunks, 'little and often!' for 15 to 20 minutes daily.

Session eight

- Revision of the early sessions is again quite brief, but a few minutes are spent on the floor revising first Accent bounce and 3/4 patterns both in semi-supine and side lying positions.

- Some work with movement, including swaying both side-by-side and face-to-face, arm and leg movements in 3/4 and marching in 4/4, is carried out.

- 3/4 patterns are practised, sitting, with syllable babble. Any consonant is combined with any vowel. By this stage the airflow and connections achieved with fricatives should be carried into other consonant sounds. Stops, glides and nasals are all used and with any monothong vowel or diphthong. Vowels and consonants may now vary within a single rhythmic pattern.

146

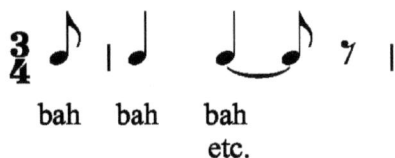

bah   bah   bah
etc.

Study patterns 3/4 babble with any consonant

- 4/4 patterns are practised, sitting, with fricative babble, similar to that used in 3/4.

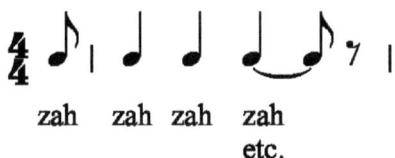

zah zah zah zah
etc.

Study Patterns 4/4 Fricative Babble

- Some complex rhythmic patterns are practised, releasing onto vowel sounds from voiced fricatives.

- Cool down is carried out as before.

- Connection into singing continues with the octave syllable exercises extended by repeating the scale, as per Janice Chapman's instructions (see Chapter 9.

- Glides and semi-occluded vocal tract exercises are practised over more extended ranges (i.e., the 9th).

- The 15–20 minute daily practice rule continues to apply.

Session nine

- A brief revision of the floor work is carried out.

- Swaying both side-by-side and face-to-face is practised with single fricatives and with first Accent Bounce.

- Release from a voiced fricative to vowels is also introduced during the side-by-side swaying.

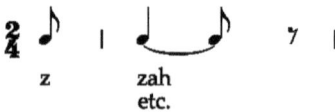

Study Patterns 1st Accent Bounce Release to Vowels

- Practice of arm, leg and body movements continues, with patterns in both 3/4 and 4/4 tempi.

- While standing, work with arms extended, shoulder height, elbows bent. This maintains the appropriate, slightly elevated, chest posture throughout the whole breath cycle. This exercise develops rapid flexible in-breaths that do not disturb the overall singing posture.

- Sitting in the chair, all the patterns are practised with consonant and vowel syllable babble. 3/4 and 4/4 are also practised with exclamations (words or short phrases that match the patterns of accentuation).

Study Patterns Exclamations

- Cool down as before.

- Connection to singing exercises continues as described above.

- The daily practice regime is continued.

Session ten

- No new work is added in this final session.

- All patterns are practised with syllable babble. The 3/4 and 4/4 patterns with exclamations are also practised.

- Isolated vowel sounds and pitch intonations are also integrated into some of the patterns.

- All forms of movement exercises are revised to ensure that the student is able to use the correct breathing pattern in a variety of postures and situations.

- Cool down occurs as before.

- Connection into singing exercises is carried out as for Session Nine.

- At this final session, students are reminded to include Accent Method exercises as part of their daily warm-up routine. After all, the Accent Method is for life not just for Christmas! A 15– 20 minute session of Accent Method practice each day should continue for ever and ever and ever.

Bibliography

References

Agostoni, E. and Sant'Amrogio, G. (1970) The diaphragm. In: E.M.J. Campbell, E. Agsotoni & J. Newsom Davis *The Respiratory Muscles Mechanics and Neural Control* (pp. 145–160). Philadelphia, PA and London: W.B. Saunders Company.

Bassiouny, S. (1998) Efficacy of the accent method of voice therapy. *Folia Phoniatrica et Logopaedica, 50,* 146–164.

Bouhuys, A., Proctor, D.F. and Mead, J. (1966) Kinetic aspects of singing. *Journal of Applied Physiology, 21,* 483–496.

Brown, W.E. (1957). *Vocal Wisdom (Enlarged Edition) Maxims of Giovanni Battista Lamperti.* New York, NY: Talpinger Publishing Company.

Bunch, M.A. (1997) *Dynamics of the Singing Voice* 4edn. New York, NY: Springer-Verlag.

Campbell, E.J.M. (1970) Accessory muscles. In: E.M.J. Campbell, E. Agsotoni & J. Newsom Davis *The Respiratory Muscles Mechanics and Neural Control* (pp. 181–193). Philadelphia, PA and London: W.B. Saunders Company

Campbell, E.M.J. and Newsom Davis, J. (1970) The intercostal muscles and other muscles of the rib cage. In E.M.J. Campbell, E. Agsotoni & J. Newsom Davis *The Respiratory Muscles Mechanics and Neural Control* (pp. 161–174). Philadelphia, PA and London: W.B. Saunders Company

Chapman, J.C. (2006) *Singing and Teaching Singing – A Holistic Approach to Classical Voice.* San Diego, CA: Plural Publishing, Inc.

Chapman, J.C. (2012) *Singing and Teaching Singing – A Holistic Approach to Classical Voice* 2edn. San Diego, CA: Plural Publishing, Inc.

Fex, B., Fex, S., Shiromoto, O. and Hirano, M. (1994) Acoustic analysis of functional dysphonia: before and after voice therapy (Accent Method). *Journal of Voice*, 8(2), 163–167.

Hixon, T.J. (2006) *Respiratory Function in Singing. A Primer for Singers and Singing Teachers.* Tucson, AZ: Redington Brown

Hixon, T.J. (1987) *Respiratory Function in Speech and Song.* Boston, MA: College-Hill Press.

Kotby, M.N. (1995) *The Accent Method of Voice Therapy.* San Diego, CA: Singular Publishing Group, Inc.

Leonard, C.H. (1983) *The Concise Gray's Anatomy.* Ware: Omega Books Ltd.

Leanderson, R. and Sundberg, J. (1988) Breathing for singing. *Journal of Voice*, 2(1), 212.

McKinney, J.C. (1994) *The Diagnosis and Correction of Vocal Faults: A Manual for Teachers of Singing and Choir Directors.* Nashville, TN: Genevox Music Group.

Miller, R. (1986) *The Structure of Singing: System and Art in Vocal Technique* New York, NY: Wadsworth.

Miller, R. (2000) *Training Soprano Voices.* New York, NY: Oxford University Press.

Proctor, D.F. (1980) *Breathing, Speech and Song.* New York, NY: Springer-Verlag.

Reynolds, S.A. (2005) *Virtual Sax Lesson – Breathing.* Retrieved July 17, 2005, from http://home.jps.net/~bflat7/breath.html.

Rubin, J.S. (1998) Mechanism of respiration (the bellows) In: Harris, T., Harris, S., Rubin, J.S. and Howard, D.M. *The Voice Clinic Handbook* (pp. 49–63). London: Whurr Publishers.

Sundberg, J. (1987) *The Science of the Singing Voice* Dekalb, Il: Northern Illinois University Press.

Sundberg, J., Leanderson, R., von Euler, C. and Knutsson, E. (1991) Influence of body posture and lung volume on subglottal pressure control during singing. *Journal of Voice*, 5(4), 283–291.

Thorpe, C.W., Cala, S.J., Chapman, J. and Davis, P.J. (2001) Patterns of breath support in projection of the singing voice. *Journal of Voice*, 15(1), 86–104.

Thurman, L. (2004) Myth-conceptions? About breathing for singing and speaking. *Australian Voice, 10,* 28–37.

Thyme-Frøkjær, K. and Frøkjær-Jenson, B. (2001) *The Accent Method: A Rational Voice Therapy in Theory and Practice.* Bicester: Speechmark Publishing Ltd.

Vennard, W. (1967) *Singing: The Mechanism and the Technic.* New York, NY: Carl Fisher Inc.

Watson, P.J. and Hixon, T.J. (1985) Respiratory kinematics in classical (opera) singers. *Journal of Speech and Hearing Research, 28,* 104–122.

Watson, P.J. and Hixon, T.J. (!987) Respiratory kinematics in classical (opera) singers. In: Hixon, T.J. *Respiratory Function in Speech and Song.* Boston, MA: College-Hill Press.

Watson, P.J., Hixon, T.J., Strathopoulos, E.T. and Sullivan, D.R. (1990) Respiratory kinematics in female classical singers. *Journal of Voice, 4*(2), 120–128.

Watson, P.J., Hoit, J.D., Lansing, R.W. and Hixon, T.J. (1989) Abdominal muscle activity during classical singing. *Journal of Voice, 3*(1), 24–31.

White, R.C. (1988) On the teaching of breathing for the singing voice. *Journal of Voice, 2*(1), 26–29.

Suggested additional reading

Blades-Zeller, E. (2002) *A Spectrum of Voices: Prominent American Voice Teachers Discuss the Teaching of Singing.* Lanham, MD: The Scarecrow Press Inc.

Boone, D.R. (1983). *The Voice and Voice Therapy.* Englewood Cliffs, NJ: Prentice-Hall Inc.

Bunch, M.A. (1998) *A Handbook of the Singing Voice.* London: Meribeth Bunch

Burgin, J.C. (1973) *Teaching Singing.* Metuchen, NJ: The Scarecrow Press Inc.

Caldwell, R. and Wall, J. (2001) *Excellence in Singing: Multilevel Learning and Multilevel Teaching.* Redmond, WA: Caldwell Publishing Company.

Colton, R.H. and Estill J. (1981) Elements of voice quality: perceptual, acoustic and physiologic aspects. In: N.J. Lass (Ed) *Speech and Language: Advances in Basic Research and Practice* (vol. V). New York, NY: Academic Press.

Coffin, B. (1989) *Historical Vocal Pedagogical Classics.* London: The Scarecrow Press Inc.

De Alcantara, P. (1997) *Indirect Procedures: A Musician's Guide to the Alexander Technique.* Oxford: Oxford University Press.

Emmons, S. (1988) Breathing for Singing. *Journal of Voice, 2*(1), 30–35.

Foulds-Elliott, S.D., Thorpe, C.W., Cala, S.J. and Davis, P.J. (2000) Respiratory function in operatic singing: effects of emotional connection. *Logopedics Phoniatrics Vocology, 25,* 151–168.

Fromkin, V., Rodman, R. and Hyams, N. (1998) *An Introduction to Language.* Orlando, FL: Harcourt Brace College Publishers.

Garcia, M. (1984) *A Complete Treatise on the Art of Singing: Part One.* New York, NY: Da Capo Press.

Harris, S. (1998). Speech therapy for dysphonia. In: Harris, T., Harris, S., Rubin, J. S. and Howard, D.M., *The Voice Clinic Handbook* (pp. 139–206). London: Whurr Publishers.

Heinrich, N. (2006) Mirroring the voice: from Garcia to the present day: some insights into singing voice registers. *Logopedics Phoniatrics Vocology, 31*(1), 3–14.

Hixon T.J. and Hoit, J.D. (2005) *Evaluation and Management of Speech Breathing Disorders: Principles and Methods.* Tucson, AZ: Redington Brown.

Hixon, T.J., Watson, P.J., Harris, F.P. and Pearl, N.B. (1988) Relative volume changes of the rib cage and abdomen during prephonatory chest wall posturing. *Journal of Voice, 2*(1), 13–19.

Husler, F. and Rodd-Marling, Y. (1960) *Singing: The Physical Nature of the Vocal Organ.* London: Faber and Faber.

Iwarsson, J. (2001) Effects of abdominal wall movement on vertical laryngeal position during phonation. *Journal of Voice, 15*(3), 384–394.

Kotby, M.N., Shiromoto, O. and Hirano, M. (1993) The Accent Method of voice therapy: effect of accentuations on FO, SPL, and airflow. *Journal of Voice, 7*(4), 319–325.

Lehman, L. (1993) *How to Sing.* New York, NY: Dover Publications Inc.

Pannbacker, M. (1998) Voice treatment techniques: a review and recommendations for outcome studies. *American Journal of Speech-Language Pathology, 7*(3), 49–64.

Pettersen, V., Bjørkøy, K., Torp, H. and Westgaard, R.H. (2005) Neck and shoulder muscle activity and thorax movement in singing and speaking tasks with variation in vocal loudness and pitch. *Journal of Voice, 19*(4), 623–34.

Pettersen, V. and Westgaard, R.H. (2004) Muscle activity in professional classical singing: a study on muscles in the shoulder, neck and trunk. *Logopedics Phoniatrics Vocology, 29,* 56–65.

Sataloff, R.T. (1998) *Vocal Health and Pedagogy* San Diego, CA: Singular Publishing Group, Inc.

Schutte, H.K. and Miller, R. (1984) Breath management in repeated vocal onset. *Folia Phoniatrica et Logopaedica, 36,* 225–232.

Shewell, C. (2009) *Voice Work: Art and Science in Changing Voices.* Chichester: Wiley-Blackwell.

Smith, S. and Thyme, K. (1976) Statistic research on changes in speech due to pedagogic treatment (The Accent Method). *Folia Phoniatrica et Logopaedica, 28,* 19–103.

Sonninen, A., Laukkanen, A-M., Karma, K. and Hurme, P. (2005) Evaluation of support in singing. *Journal of Voice 19*(2), 223–37.

Sutherland, Dame Joan, *Microsoft® Encarta® Online Encyclopedia 2005,* Retrieved July, 17, 2005, from http://encarta.msn.com © 1997–2005 Microsoft Corporation.

Thomasson, M. and Sundberg, J. (1999) Consistency of phonatory breathing patterns in professional operatic singers. *Journal of Voice, 13*(4), 529–541.

Thomasson, M. and Sundberg, J. (2001) Consistency of inhalatory breathing patterns in professional operatic singers. *Journal of Voice, 15*(3), 373–383.

Thurman, L. and Welch, G. (Eds.) (1999) *Bodymind and Voice: Foundations of Voice Education.* Fairview, MN: The Voice Care Network.

Tommasini, A. (1997, September 15) Maria Callas: A voice and a legend that still fascinate. *New York Times.* Retrieved July 17, 2005, from http://www.serendipity.li/callas/tomm.html.

About the Authors

Ron Morris, PhD

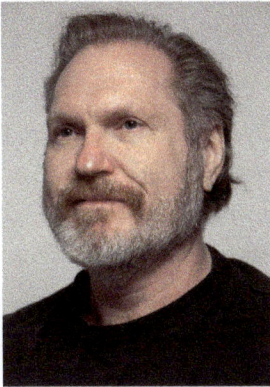

Ron Morris graduated from the University of Queensland in 1985 with a Bachelor of Speech Therapy degree. Honours in Audiology were awarded in 1986. He obtained a Masters of Music Studies degree in vocal performance in 2000 and was awarded a Doctor of Philosophy degree in Music in 2013. Ron has combined a long career (over 30 years) in Speech Therapy and Audiology with work as a professional singer.

Dr Morris is Practice Director and Senior Speech Pathologist and Audiologist at Brisbane Speech and Hearing Clinic and has special interest in working with deaf and hearing impaired clients, and with head and neck surgery and voice patients. A recognized expert in the Accent Method of breathing which is used in both voice therapy and singing, Ron is also Lecturer in Vocal Pedagogy and Vocal Health at the Queensland Conservatorium, Griffith University, Brisbane, and at the Guildhall School of Music and Drama in London.

Ron has contributed to a number of published works, including *Singing and Teaching Singing: A Holistic Approach to Classical Voice* by Janice Chapman (Plural, 3ed, 2017) and *Teaching Singing in the 21st Century* by Scott Harrison and Jessica O'Bryan (Springer, 2014).

Linda Hutchison

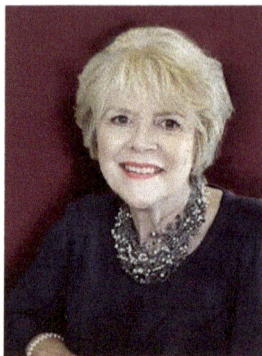

Linda Hutchison is a singing teacher, lecturer and vocal rehabilitation coach involved in the multi-disciplinary world of voice.

In her teaching practice, she works with a wide range of professionals from the classical, music theatre and jazz worlds. She is a member of the Vocal Staff at her Alma Mater, the Guildhall School of Music and Drama in London where she works with both singers and actors. She is an international guest tutor for the Irish College of Music Theatre, Dublin.

Her work in voice clinics began in 1997, which is when she first started working with the Accent Method. For five years she was a member of the Sidcup Voice Clinic at Queen Mary's Hospital in the UK and now is the Vocal Rehabilitation Coach at the Lewisham Voice Clinic, University Hospital Lewisham, London.

Alongside workshops and masterclasses, Linda gives many presentations dealing with the anatomy, physiology and care of the voice. She has created and directed professional development courses which balance the science of the voice with artistic freedom.

As a performer, her operatic career started at the age of fourteen when she sang the role of Belinda in an open air production of Purcell's Dido and Aeneas. She began her professional career as a principal soprano of the D'Oyly Carte Opera Company, later freelancing in solo operatic, concert and oratorio work. A biography of her, *Enchantment, Surely*, was published in 2010 in Tony Joseph's D'Oyly Carte Personalities series (Bunthorne Books, 2010).

Linda has been President of the British Voice Association, having been for many years a member of its Education Working Party and has served on the Council of the UK's Association of Teachers of Singing.

www.ingramcontent.com/pod-product-compliance
Ingram Content Group UK Ltd.
Pitfield, Milton Keynes, MK11 3LW, UK
UKHW022207210525
458800UK00004B/36

9 781909 082168